Saints or Quacks?

*An Exposition of the Good and the Bad of the History,
Education, and Practice of Chiropractic*

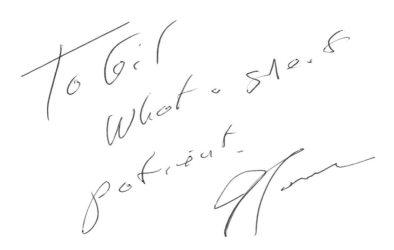

Norman Ross, B.S., D.C.

PAGE PUBLISHING, INC.
Conneaut Lake, PA

First originally published by Page Publishing 2020

ISBN 978-1-6624-0383-5 (pbk)
ISBN 978-1-6624-0384-2 (digital)

Printed in the United States of America

Contents

Foreword

Norm Ross has done it. He has given us an expository book on the art and practice of chiropractic gleaned from nearly sixty years in the profession—nearly half of chiropractic's lifespan.

He and his lovely wife have maintained a large straight chiropractic practice like some of the greats such as Jim Sigafoose, Dick Baird, and Joe Stuckey for over fifty years. This vast chiropractic experience plus the fact that he was originally educated as a school teacher and that he not only sat on two chiropractic school boards but chaired one for ten years which gave him a forward vision that no one else has seen regarding our chiropractic educational system.

In his book, Norm lays bare the scientific methodology utilized in our schools to make very good diagnosticians but drives the importance of manual adjusting the subluxation right out of our graduates, leaving many of them marginal adjustors at best. Ask many of the current technique seminar instructors, and they will tell you how unimpressed they are with our doctors' hand skills. To quote Norm, "Once you give a patient a medical diagnosis, there are no chiropractic procedures listed in the medical books to treat this person." This becomes an unattainable situation for both our patients and the profession.

When BJ Palmer was teaching straight chiropractic, we had thirty thousand chiropractors in the United States. Now that we have scientifically educated our doctors out of adjusting for decades, we have only seventy thousand licensed DCs (how many are actually still practicing?) with over 200 million more citizens! We are only seeing 5 ½ percent of the population! Forget all the therapies, pillows, and weight loss plans you are hustling on your patients and get back to adjusting them—that's why they came to you, for an adjustment!

I invite my fellow chiropractors to come along with Norm as he explains how to combine the past and the future in our educational system to enhance chiropractic presence in the world and begin to adjust a great majority of its population.

I also invite current and prospective patients to read this book and to then give it to your family and friends, even your chiropractor if they don't have their own copy; I believe it will make a better chiropractic experience for all.

David Brown
Chiropractor

As painful as change can be, it often contains the seeds of growth.

—Rabbi Daniel Lapin

Introduction

This is the story of the chiropractic profession as I have observed it, lived it, and practiced it since 1964. It is a sad story because chiropractic has so much to offer the world, yet it is not producing. It could be the answer to much pain and suffering existing today. Regrettably, the profession spends its time dealing with rules and regulations imposed by government agencies and insurance companies. The focus of these entities is more on their financial well-being than on your health and welfare.

Ever since I have been in this profession, it has tried to become something that it is not. Chiropractic has worked so hard to impress financial entities that it has lost the vision of chiropractic. I am sure most of you have heard the saying "Trying to make a silk purse out of a sow's ear." Old-timers used this saying when they saw a person or organization trying to place value on something that was not there, which is the chiropractic profession in a nutshell. It strives to deliver a product that is expensive and cannot provide any guarantee of a result because it is an intangible.

Today's chiropractor wants you to purchase this silk purse. When you go to a chiropractor's office, you enter with a hope and a prayer that good things are going to happen. Eighty percent of the time, great things do happen—when you get your hips aligned, your sacrum leveled, and your spine adjusted. The fantastic thing about chiropractic is that a chiropractor can help you using only their hands and their knowledge. They do not need fancy equipment or gadgets to give you relief. A chiropractor can be blind or deaf yet are still able to adjust and correct subluxations without having to see or hear you. It is incredible what chiropractors can do using only their hands to make you feel better.

When you go to a chiropractor hoping for results, the only thing that has happened is the chiropractor moved part of your structure from point B, where it was out of place, to point A, where it is back in its proper position. The chiropractor gives you nothing tangible to take home for the fee you paid. You go out the door as you came in, with a hope and prayer that the adjustment is going to make you feel better. It has been my observation over the past fifty-plus years of practicing chiropractic that 80 percent of the time, patients leave feeling better as the result of being adjusted.

You may be asking, "Well, Norm, if you say the results are this outstanding, why aren't 80 percent of the population going to the chiropractor?" The answer is the "aspirin bottle and a six-pack." Many chiropractors charge what *they* think *they* are worth, and they disregard what the patient can afford or is willing to pay out of their pocket for an intangible service. There is a tipping point as to how much someone will pay to become pain-free. If the price is too high, the "aspirin bottle and the six-pack" win out.

This then becomes the dilemma of the chiropractic profession. It wants to receive high fees like their counterparts, the medical doctors (medics), but how can they compete? What can they do? How can they pull in high fees? Well, that is where my fellow chiropractors have done their utmost to make a silk purse out of a plain old sow's ear.

For this reason, I, Norm Ross, a chiropractor who loves being a chiropractor, am willing to call a vast majority of my colleagues quacks—not just quacks but super quacks! However, before my fellow chiropractors get too upset with me, let me explain. There is a perception, mainly spread by the medical community, that chiropractors are quacks. Medical organizations and affiliates are the major promoters of this myth; however, chiropractic schools are complicit in fostering this idiom by graduating doctors of chiropractic medicine and chiropractic physicians instead of chiropractors. The attempt to duplicate and ape the medical profession is one of the more significant reasons the perception of quack follows us. If chiropractors would stick to their specialty, be available to give everyone a spinal adjustment when they need it using their skills and abilities, the tag of quack could quickly become saint or super saint. How about that—going from quack, cultist, or charlatan to a saint! The beauty is that this can happen. Guess who would benefit. Sure, it would help chiropractors, but the public would be the greatest benefactor.

No one likes to be the butt end of a slur. The beautiful thing is, the chiropractic profession does not have to be relegated to quacks; they do have the potential of being a saint.

However, the profession will have to step up and make some significant changes where needed, which would not be difficult to execute and administer. The profession has everything in place to quickly rectify what is wrong, and these changes need to be implemented not for the sake of the chiropractor but for everyone's benefit. Unfortunately, chiropractic is seeing only 5 percent of the population, which keeps many deserving people from receiving the great benefits that chiropractic has to offer. There's no need for chiropractors to be called quacks, cultists, and charlatans. The profession does not need to be treated like second-class citizens or closet cases when, with a few changes, we could all be saints.

Presently the profession suffers because chiropractors were maliciously labeled as quacks by the AMA. Chiropractic is a minority in the health-care field. When you belong to a minority, there will always be disparaging remarks made toward those who do not conform to the status quo. There has been bullying since time began. We used to play king of the hill, where you tried to shove the bully off the top of the hill. In health care, medics are the king, and they are the bullies.

The chiropractic profession has always existed in the shadow of the medical king of the hill. Before 1987, medical school textbooks taught that chiropractors were to be called quacks, charlatans, cultists, and rabid mad dog killers.[1] It was only by a Federal Court order that this practice was stopped.

---

[1] *Guilty*, A document produced by The Motion Palpation Institute, (Huntington Beach, California).

Editorial note: This book has been a work in progress for the last thirty-two years. We realize research has produced exciting results proving the chiropractic theory since that time. This manuscript has been left in its original form for continuity.

Chiropractors are shunned. There was a period after 1987 that the shunning subsided, but lately, it has picked up in earnest. Interestingly, we are finding that female medical doctors are the ones most vocal about not wanting their patients utilizing chiropractic care. I presume it is because women medics have the dilemma of competing with their male counterparts. They possibly feel competition with arrogant medical males is enough, and they do not want chiropractors giving them additional competition.

The chiropractic profession should have cinched their bootstraps, thumbed their nose at the medical profession, told the insurance industry to "shove it," and concentrated on helping more people in this suffering world. Had we done this, we wouldn't be on the outside looking in. We would become competitive and could be seeing close to 80 percent of the population.

It is a sad story for a great profession that has been around for 125 years yet sees only 5 percent of the population. These are statistics for the US, and it is much less in the rest of the world. How regretful its educational system was set up by legislative bodies at the instigation of the medical profession and which has not yet changed to benefit the profession or patients. Sadly, chiropractors manage patient care according to insurance protocol rather than the actual need of the patient. How sorrowful it is that the chiropractic profession has become out of touch regarding its mission, purpose, and responsibility to society.

Pain is devastating when it penetrates an individual's lifestyle, productivity, and leisure activities. Unfortunately, in today's health-care world, primarily, the only answer to solve this dilemma is pills, pills, and more pills. The chiropractic profession has a method that can alleviate many of the problems of the working world. What a boon to America and the world if chiropractors saw 50 to 95 percent of the world's population instead of a mere 5 percent.

The purpose of this book is to inform the public that everyone should and could have access to affordable chiropractic care and also to rekindle the chiropractors' vision of how they can provide readily available chiropractic care to all humankind. Another goal is to motivate the chiropractic colleges to revise their curriculum and direct the courses studied, thus enabling their graduates to be qualified experts with the skill and excitement to care for 95 percent of the population, therefore helping to alleviate the health-care crisis in our country and proclaim the benefit of chiropractic to the public.

The beautiful song "He's Got the Whole World in His Hands" makes a statement. God does have the whole world in his hands. Chiropractors have been taught an incredible skill utilizing their hands and can truly become an extension of God. Chiropractors do have the whole world in God's and their hands if they only knew it.

Please read this book, give it to your friends, neighbors, coworkers, and please give it to your chiropractor. Tell the world what chiropractic should be and what it should be doing. It is about you and your family's future, as to whether you will be able to receive health care that can make a difference in all your lives. Encourage your kids to go to chiropractic school. With your help, we can make this world a better place.

CHAPTER 1

The Long Life of Uncle Gene

I checked in on my uncle late one night—he was sleeping peacefully. I sat down beside him and started writing in my book. It was serene, with a soft, warm August breeze wafting through the room. The soffit lights reflected around the edges of the ceiling, giving a gentle glow like the sun radiating off the clouds as it slips over the horizon. Relaxing religious instrumental music played in the background. Uncle Gene, with his full head of white hair and in his white gown, lay relaxed on the white bed with white bed sheets. It was angelic, a peaceful situation that I wished would go on forever.

My spell broke as a nurse quietly slipped into the room and gently asked how he was doing. I described what a comfortable fifteen minutes I had enjoyed. She went over to check on him, and after an examination, she said, "I'll get another nurse. I don't think he's with us!"

Uncle Gene was ninety-nine and one half years old when he passed on an August night in 2003. He had a long, productive life, with minimal health problems and had only taken ill the day before. I sat with him that night and knew that old age and not outside or traumatic factors were causing him to slip away. Earlier in the day, he wanted to know what the price of corn and soybean futures were for the day. He never gave up; he was still trying to make money on the day of his death. If asked how he was, he would say, "Just wonderful." Uncle Gene never dwelled on his problems; instead, he always asked about others. "How are you doing? Are you making any money? How are you going to pay your taxes?" He maintained a zest for life right up to the afternoon of his death.

Dr. Reggie Gold, a well-known chiropractic philosopher, speaks of life being like a candle. A candle lit on one end should burn to the bottom, flicker once or twice, and go out. Uncle Gene's life was like that candle; he flickered the day of his death and passed peacefully that evening. I sat in his room for about an hour after the funeral director had taken his body away, quietly reflecting on his life and wondering why everyone could not have good health and long life that he possessed. He had a sound mind, was able to read a newspaper with nonprescription reading glasses, and kept up on current events at the age of ninety-nine! Why was he so different from the average man? Statistics show that the American male lives on an average of 76.1 years.[2] Life is a struggle for many people in the golden years. My question that night was, what made Uncle Gene's life so vibrant and long? Why did his candle burn down to the bottom without sputtering and going out long before its time?

Uncle Gene's parents lived to ages eighty and ninety. He never had a demanding job. His surroundings were comfortable; he always had food on the table and never had detrimental stress. I thought, *Yes if everyone lived in that type of environment, all could live to the age of ninety-nine.* Well, maybe not. We know that statistically, there are people who have everything and who also die at the average age of seventy-six years old. Money to purchase cars, homes, and boats does not mean that you will have a long life. Authorities say, what you eat, how much exercise you get, your education, environment, sanitation, hygiene, and accessibility to doctors determine longevity. Fifteen percent of the commercials on TV and radio bombard us with how to stay healthy with drugs. It has been said that 17 percent of our gross national product is spent on health and drug care to make us healthier and happier. Men are only living an average of 76.1 years and women 81.1 years when scientists say the body is capable of living to the age of 150.

There is one thing that Uncle Gene did throughout his life that roughly only 5 percent of the population does concerning their health.

[2]   National Center for Health Statistics, United States, 2017: With special feature on mortality. Hyattsville, MD. 2018

It has been around for 125 years. It is mostly known through word of mouth and possibly helps more people with health problems than anyone can imagine, even though only a fraction of the population utilizes it. It helps the labor force keep moving every day. Without it, lost time on the job would be tremendous and the cost of goods and services would be much higher. It is a profession that is taken for granted and even shunned. It is a profession that leaves no scars; it is a profession without a face. It is the chiropractic profession. Estimates state that only 5 percent of the population of the United States goes to chiropractors. Gene was one of that 5 percent. Uncle Gene's use of this profession throughout his life is what helped him live longer and die peacefully. He believed that when you got "out of fix," you went to the chiropractor.

Chiropractic was founded in 1895 in Davenport, Iowa, nine years before Uncle Gene was born in February of 1904. Because of his interest in reading, back in the 1920s, he came across some of the early writings of BJ Palmer, the developer of chiropractic. Immediately upon reading Palmer's ideas of health, Gene could comprehend the simple application of those principles.

As a result, he embraced those concepts as a way to keep and maintain good health, and he continued that commitment until his death. As I look back at that night, I am sure that being adjusted when he needed it was a major reason he lived twenty-three and a half years longer than the average male.

The spinal adjustments that Uncle Gene received periodically are quite simple. They are not much different than straightening the handlebars on your bicycle when they get bent or straightening the front of your car when it gets out of alignment. Uncle Gene functioned better when he was in adjustment.

There has to be an order in all things that move and function. There has to be resistance for movement and function to take place. The simple concept that the Palmers observed, that no one else in medicine was paying attention to, was structure. When the structure is misaligned, what effect does that misalignment have on the health of the body? The medical field concentrates on the chemical and traumatic aspects of health. The structural and functional integrity of the body and its relationship to health were not addressed until DD and BJ Palmer came along with their observations and theories. Some say that AT Still, the founder of osteopathy, beat the Palmers in saying that structure played a role in health care. Today, osteopaths have pretty much given up on addressing the structural part of health care because it is more lucrative and easier to dispense pills.

Uncle Gene was similar to a machine that is affected by our greatest enemy—gravity and resistance. For anything to move, there has to be resistance. Bearings have to be tight and snug around an axle for the wheel to move correctly. Pistons need to be close fitting in the cylinders for the gas to explode correctly in the chamber without leakage so the engine will run efficiently. In the body, each joint has to have resistance against it. When energy explodes in the muscle, the body propels forward. Uncle Gene had an understanding of these unforeseen forces that rule our lives. He began using chiropractic to keep his body in alignment. Whenever he had stress or discomfort, which did not correct itself after a couple of days, Uncle Gene would then visit Old Doc Shay. After an adjustment or two, he would be "back in the pink," as he would say. I became a licensed chiropractor in 1968. Shortly after that, Old Doc Shay passed away, and Uncle Gene asked me to check his alignment and adjust him. I did this for him for the next thirty-five years.

Was keeping him structurally in adjustment the only reason he lived ninety-nine and a half years with remarkable agility, very little pain, a healthy positive attitude and setting goals up to his death? No, but it did play a huge role. When people have joint pain or chronic pain, it eventually overwhelms what they think about all day. Their mind becomes obsessed with the discomfort and on how they can rid themselves of this albatross. Uncle Gene had none of this. He was an example of longevity and the importance of chiropractic care.

One of the main reasons I am a chiropractor is to offer you something you are not going to receive from other health-care providers. My job is to restore and maintain the structural integrity of the body, to balance the hips, level the sacrum, and straighten the spine. Once the spinal structure is addressed and any unnecessary pressure is off the nerves and vessels that pass alongside, the integrity of the nervous system and blood vessels will take over and heal you. The power that made the body can and will heal the body if given a chance, provided it has no interference.

Everyone should have the right to receive chiropractic care when they need it, and everyone needs it from time to time. Chiropractic has proven to get results since its inception. It worked then, and the same principles work today. If it did not work, it would not have lasted 125 years.

I hope this book will give you new perceptions about the chiropractic profession, some of its good points and some of its not so good. Many of you are suffering and have nowhere to turn to find an answer. Chiropractic has helped millions of people who found no solution elsewhere. You should have an opportunity to have a chiropractor evaluate you to see if chiropractic can help you. I hope that you can find a chiropractor that loves to adjust and is willing to try to help all situations regardless of the condition or the financial ability to pay. There is no reason you should not have the opportunity to live a long, happy, pain-free life like my uncle Gene.

Going to the chiropractor should be a fun and easy task. Uncle Gene went to Old Doc Shay, who was quite a talker; he would tell about his days in the New York Yankees farm system. Dr. Shay was an up-and-coming baseball player and was only a season away from making the big time with the Yankees. Like many athletes, an injury occurred that laid him flat on his back for too long to get back into the baseball routine. After standard medical methods of pills, and when more pills failed, he finally went to a chiropractor. He had his hips aligned, his sacrum leveled, and his lower spine straightened, which got him back on his feet. He was so impressed with his turnaround that he decided to go to chiropractic school so he could help others who found themselves in a similar plight.

Back in the early 1900s, many students who were in chiropractic school were there because they saw what benefits it had given them. In those years, the school was eighteen months long, and tuition was low. They could pack their bags and be off to Davenport, Iowa, and in no time, they became a chiropractor. They were ready for the world, anx-

NORMAN ROSS, B.S., D.C.

ious to help all who were hurting, suffering, and not knowing where to turn for help. The new chiropractors coming out of school were excited. They wanted to help people. It was not a job to them; it was a mission!

Unfortunately, times have changed. Today chiropractors come out of school looking at treating you as a job; it is no longer a mission for many. Chiropractic schools are now five years in length following a two-year general college prerequisite, for a total of seven years. It is a lot tougher getting a chiropractic degree today than it was in Dr. Shay's time. All the school appeared to need then was a warm, upright body that could pay the tuition. Students today are running up enormous tuition debts for seven years of classwork. Some of that money went for living expenses, which allow students to live high on the hog while in school. Since graduates are coming out of school with massive debt, their attitude has changed. Chiropractic is no longer a mission as it was for Dr. Shay, but a job requiring a lot of work and high fees to pay off an enormous debt.

It might be a while before you find the likes of a compassionate, caring, and talkative Dr. Shay. Because of computer technology, social media, paperless records, etc., chiropractors have become more sophisticated than Dr. Shay. Today, many chiropractors diagnose you on the computer versus palpating and examining you, and they adjust you with handheld computer-driven equipment. Very few use their hands, as Dr. Shay did. They also use insurance procedures; they know all the right codes to get paid high fees. Dr. Shay did everything in cash. He never sent a bill to anyone, and he never worried about being paid, but he always was! Today, most chiropractors will make you sign a note to guarantee that they will get paid. It is a much more formal atmosphere when you go into a chiropractor's office today. Rules and regulations set by entities (insurance companies and the government) are more focused on their financial well-being than on your health and welfare. The students must repay huge tuition debts. Young financially strapped chiropractors are possibly more interested in you helping them pay off their debts than they are in helping you structurally.

Until you can find a chiropractor like Dr. Shay, let me give you a home exercise that can help keep your back healthy and agile. This exer-

22 | THE LONG LIFE OF UNCLE GENE

cise is the shower squat. If you do it every day, you will see a remarkable difference in the way your back feels. What is unique about this is that it does not require you to wallow around on the floor. It will not take an additional minute out of your busy schedule as other exercises do. Pretty cool, eh!

SHOWER EXERCISE

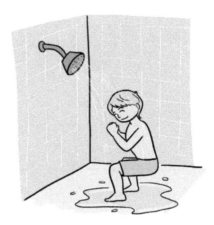

1. Get in the shower, lather up, rinse off in a squatting position.
2. Rinsing off is actually boring. Let's put this time to good use.
3. Squatting draws the hips and knees tight. The heat and weight of the water help draw the joints tighter.
4. Do this daily and watch your structural alignment improve.

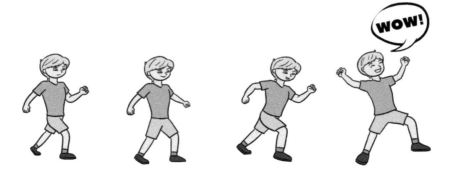

WOW!

CHAPTER 2

Humanity's Common Nemesis, Backaches!

Everyone has a backache at one time or another, and if you have never had one, you are a phenomenon, a miracle, or a downright oddity. Backaches will range from mild to severe and can be incapacitating. We have all heard horror stories, curses, and amazing cures that accompany this malady. Backaches exist—it is part of life—and it has been a problem ever since man and woman have existed.

According to evolutionists, backaches started when man emerged from the horizontal position of the animal, on to the chimp, then on to the upright position. Did you hear about the chimps that were declared humans? I believe the case was eventually overturned, but in April 2015, a judge in New York ruled that Hercules and Leo were legal persons. Hercules and Leo were laboratory chimps used in experimentation at Stony Brook College in New York. The judge "effectively recognizes the chimpanzees as legal humans."[3] I wonder if this judge might have any evidence that these chimps, or any forefather chimps, suffered from backaches. I presume they were afflicted the same as us.

If the evolutionists are right and we walked on four legs, we possibly would have less back pain. The spinal vertebra of four-legged animals is essentially the same as ours. However, the effects of gravity are markedly different as it forces more compression on our upright spine.

---

[3] Mail Online by Sara Malm, April 21, 2015, https://www.dailymail.co.uk/news/article-3048579/Chimpanzees-given-HUMAN-rights-NY-judge-rules-two-primates-held-research-lab-covered-laws-govern-detention-people.html

Whether we were animals or apes, according to evolutionists or upright human beings made in God's image, our spine is a vertical pole susceptible to the forces of gravity. We have to deal with this reality daily.

To make a living today, many of our jobs require repetitive work, which, along with accidents, will cause the highest number of backaches. Habits, congenital problems, stupidity, and unforeseen circumstances can also be causes of this prevalent aggravation.

Backaches cause more work loss time than any other human affliction. Not everyone gets the big three problems (cancer, heart, and diabetes) that the media highlights, but almost everyone does or will have a backache.

When you have to deal with pain, you typically consult a medical doctor who will give you their assessment of your condition. You take their word for it because they are the authority. However, they are not always able to accurately assess you or correct your malady, so you often hear that you should have a second opinion. With this in mind, I want to demonstrate how you can check yourself at home as to whether or not you have a structural back problem. You will then be able to go to the doctor aware of structural issues, and you can tell them you have a second opinion—your own.

DAILY MIRROR CHECK

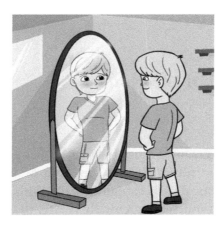

1. Before you slip into the shower and do your "shower squat," go to the mirror and check your hips.
2. Measure them to see if they are level.
3. Place your hands flat over the crest of the hips.
4. Your goal is to have level hips.
5. If one hip appears high and stays high for a number of days, that is not a good sign and it is time for you to be off to the chiropractor.

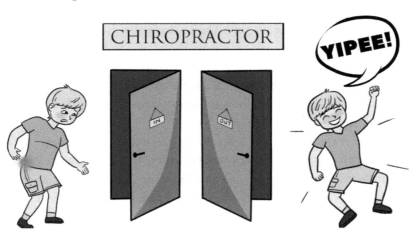

CHAPTER 3

Trouble Down the Road

What do I mean by trouble down the road? Can measuring hip height tell you about your future? It sure can. Your body's structure plays one of the most critical parts to your overall health, and knowing how to read and check yourself structurally is vital to your future health. There are two types of functions in our bodies that I want to discuss, the chemical and the structural. We are very familiar with the chemical aspects of health. Every day, we are bombarded with news and magazine articles regarding drugs. Television and radio advertisements are continually blaring out advice as to what medications we should be taking to have excellent health. According to the AMA press release on November 17, 2015, it stated that AMA calls for ban on direct to consumer advertising of prescription drugs and medical devices. In 2012, the pharmaceutical industry spent more than $27 billion on drug promotion—and more than $24 billion on marketing to physicians. They go on to say in this AMA article that because of the ads, 28 percent of the public ask for a drug they saw advertised and that 12 percent say their doctor prescribed it. I would guess that the public is well informed about the chemical aspect of health. Isn't it interesting that almost 30 percent of the population can tell their doctor what drug they think is best for them?

However, no one ever talks about the other component of the body's health equation, the structural portion. You can have the correct chemicals in the exact formulas, but if the structure is out of alignment, the body will not function as it should and pain will usually ensue.

Every day, gravity takes its toll on us and continually changes our structure. What an effort it takes for us to get up in the morning—we have to push up against the gravitational pressure that is always pressing down on us. When we make it up, we force ourselves to stay up for sixteen, seventeen, or eighteen straight hours. After all this time of being upright, we get tired and have to lie down. We stay horizontal for eight hours for our body to regroup so we can give tomorrow another eighteen hours of being upright.

One of our biggest jobs in life is staying upright. We push up against gravity that is pulling down on us. If we live to be eighty years old, that is thirty thousand days of ups and downs. In time, there is a slight bit of compression that takes place every day; eventually, we will lose from two to three inches of height in those eighty years.

By the time we go to bed at night, we will be one half to three fourths of an inch shorter than when we got up in the morning. You can measure and see for yourself. Loss of height or shrinkage is caused by fluid contained in our vertebral discs being squashed out of these fibers by the weight of our body. The disc is the cushion or donut between the vertebra. During sleep, the discs fill with fluid so that when you get up in the morning, you will have regained the one half to three fourths of an inch you lost yesterday.

Now for the exciting part. During the night's rest and the refilling of the fluid, if there are vertebral misalignments that have occurred during the day, your body has the innate wisdom to reset or readjust the vertebrae. How awesome is that! Let's say you were out playing with the kids and you tripped over a fallen tree branch; you went down pretty hard on your hip and also jarred your right arm as you tried to stop your fall. Oh, it wasn't much; you jump up, brush yourself off, shake it out, and go back to playing. Later in the day, you began noticing stiffness in your shoulder. It was somewhat annoying, but not bad. When you got up the next morning, there were no problems or any discomfort. Isn't it fantastic how the body can rectify problems? I am sure all of you have experienced this phenomenon time and again. You feel tough before you go to bed, and through the night, magic happens. And voila, the next morning, you are fine. This is an experience we all have had, but we take it for granted.

Seldom do we ever consider what happened through the night. We accept we will get better, and rarely does our body let us down. What happens to make us better while we snooze? Well, you have a little ol' chiropractor in you who adjusts your vertebrae—just kidding! But the vertebra and structures that were moved out of place in your fall can correct themselves. When you lie down, the discs start to refill and balloon up as you are stretched out in a horizontal position and the vertebra reposition and reset themselves back to their normal position. We have to remember we were made perfect and everything started in its proper place. However, when a vertebra becomes compromised and twisted, they do not want to stay that way. They want to return to their normal position, and they will if we give them half a chance. Unfortunately, we are the ones who screw things up—falling over limbs, slipping on spilled water, and doing repetitive activities. Remarkably, the body has this innate ability to correct itself; otherwise, we would be in big trouble.

CHAPTER 4

Structural Ranges

Joints in the body have four ranges of motion. The first is the normal range; an example is moving any joint to its maximum. The second, or auxiliary, range is moving the joint beyond its comfort zone, where it can be executed without any repercussions. The third is the reserve auxiliary, which causes strain, as when a thread starts pulling away from the stitching. The fourth is the tearing range. All the ranges are like pop-off valves, circuit breakers, or a five-mile per hour bumper. They have to be there, or an overload would create serious problems.

If falling over the downed limb caused the joint to move into the third area, the auxiliary reserve range, it may be more difficult for the body to correct itself overnight. When there is strain and tissue pull, the body automatically sends fluid to the damaged tissue for cleaning and repair, causing the area to be congested. If this traffic jam is not too severe, it may take three or four nights for the vertebrae to correct themselves.

Sometimes, resting overnight will not break a fixated joint loose. When this happens, it is time for you to look in the mirror and evaluate yourself posturally. Facing the mirror, find the hip ledges on each side of your body. Place your hands horizontally across the surface on each side with the fingers pointing toward the mirror. You are looking to see if your hands are level. If one hand is much higher than the other, check it for three or four days. There will be times that it will take multiple nights before it retracts from the auxiliary range and resolves itself.

However, there will be situations when resting will not loosen the restriction. If after several nights with your hip checks it is still showing one side much higher than the other, it is now time to start thinking about getting checked professionally. Hip bones have the right to move side to side, but when they have completed their job, they are obligated to return to their proper position. When we are driving and come upon a slowpoke, we pull out into the left lane and go around. But once around, we are obligated to return to our lane. If we stay in the passing lane, which we had the right to move into, but do not honor our responsibility of returning to our proper position, we are asking for trouble. Likewise, with the hip structure, they need to be level, or significant problems will be lurking ahead if that range of motion is not maintained.

Foretelling the Future

Yes, we can foresee some of our future by checking our hips. If the hips stay locked with one side high and the other low, one thing after another will start to take place:

1. The base of the spine or sacrum will tip.
2. The vertebrae will tilt.
3. The hips will rub and strain.
4. The ball and sockets of the hips will bind.
5. The head will try to stay upright with a compensatory tilting.

Our heads have to stay level because of the equilibrium center located behind the ears. Therefore, the ears always have to remain balanced. Because of this balancing factor, the spine has to compensate in numerous areas, which leads to problems other than structural. This adaptation of the body trying to rectify a bad situation is where degeneration of the hips and spine have their beginning.

Keeping the head level creates compensation stress points throughout the spine. These stress areas create disc bulges, or hernias; spinal degeneration; and spur formations that plague society. Unfortunately, once it gets to these stages, these conditions are challenging to correct.

Fortunately, before you get to these dangerous compensation situations, you can help yourself. Anyone who owns a car realizes they have to take it to the mechanic to have the front end aligned on occasion. Proper wheel alignment is crucial to the longevity of a vehicle, and we are no different than our vehicles. If your car gets out of alignment and you leave it out of alignment, before long, you will have to park it. You cannot drive a vehicle if the front shimmies so severely you cannot hold onto the steering wheel. When you see tire wear or you feel the shimmy, perhaps you notice a loss in gas mileage. When these things happen, off you go to the mechanic.

Comparable to the importance of proper front-end alignment in our automobile is the hip structure in our body. Just like the front end of a vehicle that takes all the abuse going down the road at 70mph, our hips take the first abuse of our daily activities. Because of this, you need to learn to check your hips to determine your alignment.

Fortunately, you can check yourself just as you check your tires. Get into the habit of standing in front of the mirror and seeing if your hips are level. It is simple and not time-consuming, but if you find they consistently stay off balance, it is time to go to the chiropractor for an aligning adjustment.

Chiropractors are skilled craftsmen. They have the knowledge and the ability to use their hands to address the structural problems of health care.

Often, chiropractic patients think we are a genius because we can palpate the spine and tell patients before they tell us where they are having problems. They will exclaim, "How did you know that!" We joke and tell them how clairvoyant we are, but in the end, we inform them that we are all built alike and that we all have the same stress points.

Stress points are usually where most of the activity of our bodies takes place. In our homes, where do we have most of our problems? Since doors, windows, or faucets get the most use, they therefore give us the most difficulties. The body is the same. We turn our head hundreds of times a day, so the middle neck vertebrae get more work than any other vertebrae in the body.

Similarly, our hips take a lot of abuse every day. Therefore, we should check them first. In chiropractic school, we study stress points over and over so we can picture every working part in those areas along with considering additional stress areas. When we get in practice, it does not take long to realize that 90 percent of all structural problems derive from five or six stress points located in our spine. So now you know that chiropractors' psychic abilities are not as extraordinary as you may have thought.

If you have never been to a chiropractor, do not be afraid. Remember, you adjust and correct yourself every night. All the chiropractor is doing is assisting you in a job your body started but cannot quite get accomplished. For example, when you go to bed feeling tough and you get up feeling better, that is how an adjustment feels. It takes the pressure off, and that is fabulous. Give chiropractic a try. You may have an 80 percent chance of feeling better, and that is pretty amazing!

CHAPTER 5

Going to the Chiropractor

Going to a chiropractor is like going to any other provider for the first time. You may be a little nervous, but be assured most people will tell you that it is a very gratifying experience. Approximately, 80 percent of patients going into the office will come out feeling better than when they went in. Stop and think about that statement. There are not many places, especially in health care, where you can go in and get that kind of help so promptly.

As a general rule of thumb, 20 percent of all chiropractic patients labor in getting better. Perhaps 20 percent of this 20 percent may not get any of the results they were seeking. Hopefully, you will take hip checking seriously and will be able to get into the approximate 80 percent group that gets good or even great results.

The chiropractor is much like a gardener. Once the seeds are planted, the ground and rainwater provide nourishment, the sun gives energy, and all we do as a gardener is keep the weeds out, and the plants upright. If we do that, the chance of having a great crop will be in the 80 percent range. However, there is a 20 percent chance of problems. The same occurs with people. Mother Nature takes care of most of our needs, but like tomatoes that sometimes have to be staked up to produce abundantly, we periodically have to be lined up to function at peak performance.

Instead of using a hoe like a gardener, the chiropractor utilizes a table and their hands. These are their tools to remove interference that will hamper growth and good health. When you first approach the chiropractor, they will want a history of how and when your problem started and where it is centered. Histories can explain as much as 80 percent of what type of adjustment the chiropractor will use to solve your problem. They will have you walk, bend, stand, sit, lie, and put you in other positions to analyze your spine, hips, and their functions. They will palpate the vertebrae, using their hands to examine and determine which way the structure has shifted. After analyzing their findings, the chiropractor will use an adjusting technique that is best suited for your situation to place the vertebrae or hips into their proper position.

Vertebrae have three arms located on its body. Each side of the vertebrae, except the front side, has an arm attached. These arms are for the attachment of muscles, but they also provide a lever for the chiropractor to use as a pry bar to lever the vertebrae back into its proper position.

The chiropractor will do most of the adjusting as you lie face down on the table. In a horizontal position, the vertebrae will pull apart, as they do at night, which allows the chiropractor to lever the subluxated vertebrae with more ease. There may be a noise or a popping sound that takes place with the adjustment, which is a vacuum sound that occurs when anything moves under pressure. Most people will say, "Wow, that felt great!" and it does. When you take the stress off of anything, it will usually feel better, like a load has lifted—what a relief.

Millions of people go to chiropractors each year. I venture to say that if an exit poll was taken as patients leave any chiropractor's office, there would be many patients stating, "I feel great, wonderful, terrific, or a heck of a lot better than when I went in." Some would say, "It's too early to tell, but some better," and a few would say, "No change" or "I feel a little worse." These are challenging cases because of acuteness, swelling, and the fact that some people just let it go too long, allowing arthritis or callus formation to set up with no hope of reversal.

Would it be worth it to go to a chiropractor when you are feeling poorly and have an 80 percent chance of feeling better and having that wow feeling? Of course, it would. Start checking your hip levels today.

The Garden

Most of us love to see a beautiful garden that is well kept, with foliage and leaves, brilliant colors, and an abundance of produce. It is a fantastic sight, whether real or in a painting, to see a bushel basket of ripe fruit piled high and overflowing.

I have painted you a picture of how the chiropractic profession could provide you and your family an overflowing abundance of good health—not having to spend 15 percent to 20 percent of your paychecks on doctors and their drugs that may treat one issue yet having the possibility of causing another much more serious problem than the original. We could use the money spent on medications for enjoyable experiences while we feel healthy, happy, and terrific as initially designed. How marvelous would that be? If people felt better, acted better, and were without pain, they would get along better. What a vision.

I have been in practice for over fifty years, and our office has seen over 150,000 different individuals who have come in as new patients. Among those numbers, there are hundreds of Uncle Gene stories. When you deal with miracles every day, as we do, they become commonplace. You do not have to take my word for it, so please visit our office. You are welcome to sit in our waiting room and ask those waiting to get an adjustment why they are coming to see Dr. Norm. Most are excited to be there and more than willing to share their stories with you. Keep track of the people you talk to and take an exit poll after they have their adjustment. Ask them questions like "What did you think of your adjustment? Did it hurt? Would you do it again? Do you think it will help you? Would you send your friend, spouse, child or boss, for an adjustment?" I will bet you the back forty that you will find almost 80 percent will be very positive.

CHAPTER 6

The Sad Story

Unfortunately, with almost every utopia, there is sure to be a fly in the ointment. In this case, it is because chiropractors want to keep a closed shop and limit the number of people they care for to a measly 5 percent of the population. Yes, that is right; only 5 percent of the US population receives the benefits of chiropractic services, and it is even less in foreign countries. Another unfortunate fact is that the people of the United States utilize 50 percent of all drugs manufactured worldwide, and the US makes up only 5 percent of the world's population. Even with all the drug usage, the US ranks seventeenth overall in health care. Can you believe those facts? We should all be outraged over these travesties. It is a crying shame.

You go to the medics and get hooked on drugs, and too many chiropractors do not want to see you for what they can do best, correct your structure. Presently, the hierarchy of the profession seeks to add prescriptive drugs to the practice of chiropractic so they too can hook more people on drugs. You have only a slim chance of being treated for your problems without a doctor pushing more pills down your throat.

The pitiful chiropractors cannot see the forest for the trees. They are so bent on being accepted by the medics and wanting to be like "real doctors" they sacrifice the public's health for their self-aggrandizement. They then turn around and wonder why they don't see more new patients. (Later in the book, I will explain why the profession only sees a small portion of the population.) As a practicing chiropractor for so many years, giving or being part of providing over one and a half million adjustments and seeing positive results from those adjustments, there is no reason we should be peddling drugs to become accepted.

Chiropractors should be giving life-restoring adjustments as described. If they did, their patients would be sending them ten or twelve new patients every day. If that is not acceptable, then I do not know what is.

What a crying shame that chiropractors sit on their talented hands and reject the masses. Then they spend time and money lobbying the authorities to allow them to help drug up the country even more than the medics have already accomplished. The chiropractic profession has a great ability to help everyone feel and act better, and we should not reject the masses to dispense more drugs. The world needs *level hips and straight spines*, not more drugs!

CHAPTER 7

Health Care or Drug Care

Upward of 20 percent of our gross national product in the US is currently spent on health care; actually, we should say drug care. There are nearly eight hundred thousand medics in the country who typically treat approximately 20 percent of the population, which uses almost 80 percent of the government and insurance health/drug care money. That is right, 20 percent of the people use 80 percent of the insurance money. That means that the rest of us pay for 20 percent of the gross national product that feeds the monsters, the federal health-care programs and private insurance industries. The mass of working people has to pay the freight that allows the medics to charge outlandish fees for 20 percent of the population. These 20 percent have learned how to work the system. Today, patients routinely come to our office with twenty prescriptions; yes, I said twenty—occasionally even more. According to Stastista.com, prescriptions per capita in the US in 2013 by age group are as follows: age groups fifty to sixty prescribed 19.2; sixty-five to seventy-nine prescribed 27.3; eighty and up, 29.1; fifty- to eighty-year-olds prescribed 19–29 prescriptions per person. It is unbelievable!

When I was a student in chiropractic school in the midsixties, and this was true of medical students as well, blood pressure readings were taught to be a person's age plus one hundred. That formula was used for years until the drug companies got into the business of selling drugs to make money for their shareholders versus giving drugs to help patients become healthy. In 1978, drug companies went public. If you and I bought a $1,000 worth of stock in the Merck Drug Company as an

investment, we would want to earn 10 percent. Drug companies strug-
gled to make money for the first few years. To remedy that problem,
in 1988, the old blood-pressure formula of age plus one hundred was
changed to a definite 120/80 regardless of age.

Guess what, with everyone having to have a standard 120/80
blood pressures, blood pressure-drug sales went through the roof.
Today, anyone over the age of forty-five will generally have a blood
pressure topping 120/80. If you visit a medic for any problem, they will
automatically put you on blood pressure medicine. Almost 80 percent
of new patients coming into our office, definitely those forty-five and
over, will confirm that they are on at least one blood pressure medication. Lowering the blood pressure formula has made a lot of investors
rich. This reformulation worked well and has made gazillions of dollars
for the drug companies. If you check out any business newspaper that
tracks the top fifty stocks, you will see that twenty-five out of the top
fifty will be drug companies. Blood pressure readings were not the only
readings that changed to sell more medicine. Other norms for the body
were altered, like cholesterol, for example. Whether it was good for you
or not, it made a lot of cents to do it.

CHAPTER 8

Havens and Respites

Earlier I described how chiropractic could help correct the so-called national health care crisis, which is more like the national health-care rip-off. Chiropractic could also provide havens, respites, and positive outcomes for many. There have been numerous polls that show 70 percent of the population would love to try chiropractic if they had the opportunity. The public has heard how wonderful adjustments feel and how much better you operate if your hips are level and your spine is in alignment. The powers that be in the profession say we have to be like the medics to be accepted by third-party payers along with government entities that shell out big bucks and grants. Instead of having an opportunity to have the life force that flows over your nervous system restored to 100 percent by getting an adjustment, they want the chiropractors to duplicate the medical/prescription model of medicine. They would rather see the profession helping the medics peddle drugs because of the money involved. You have heard it before, "follow the money." As long as the chiropractic profession continues to want to become like the medics, the profession will continue to see only 5 percent of the population, all the while moaning, groaning, and wondering why they aren't seeing more patients. They will be going to bed night after night having the same old reoccurring dream of being an accepted chiropractic physician sitting behind a fancy desk and writing scripts all day.

There is an adage that the physician should heal thyself before trying to advise others. I feel that my years of experience have given me a tremendous amount of credibility to inform my profession of its shortfalls. Being a chiropractor for over fifty years, I have observed that our profession has and exhibits a dichotomy. Mental health is a grave matter, and I do not want to offend anyone with this diagnosis. I am at a loss as to how to describe the chiropractic profession other than having multiple personalities. In my opinion, the profession is disassociated with reality and is trying to exist in a world of being something that it is not. Chiropractic schools teach their chiropractic candidates medical procedures that pertain to the practice of medicine and then send them out and ask them to be chiropractors adjusting their patients.

With my years of experience, I have concluded that chiropractic is trying to make the preverbal "silk purse out of a sow's ear." I attended National College of Chiropractic near Chicago, where I graduated as a doctor of chiropractic. Today, the same school is called National University of Health Sciences, and it graduates doctors of chiropractic medicine. National College was medically orientated when I graduated. It was difficult to diagnosis a patient's problem and give it a medical name. There were no medically diagnosed conditions that call for a chiropractic adjustment as the primary mode of care. If it was difficult back then, how impossible is it today?

Once you give a patient a medical diagnosis, there are no chiropractic procedures listed in the medical books to treat this person. Since we had no access to drugs, we would have to conjure up some half-baked remedy because almost every medical diagnosis calls for drug therapy. Since we were unable to use drugs as the first choice of care, we would cobble some analysis/diagnosis to try to treat the patient's problem. How frustrating!

To the school's credit, they did teach us how to adjust the spine and hips. I was fortunate to have been taught by Dr. Alfred States. He loved to adjust and taught all of us to become great adjustors. Unfortunately, to the administration, adjusting was almost secondary because they wanted us to be proficient as pseudo-physicians. They took pride in their graduates discovering conditions that medical doctors missed. It was like they were training us to be great diagnosticians and one-up the medics. Regrettably, it was more of a game of "one-up-manship" than finding ways to help the patient. Because once you have made the diagnosis on the medical misdiagnosis, what do you do next? By rights, you should send that medically diagnosed patient back to the MD. What then becomes the purpose of chiropractors? Will we be honest and do that, or will we keep the patient and treat them with a makeshift alternative? Morally, this is the question.

The hierarchy of the profession then, as well as today, are trying to make our students perform a medical diagnosis routine. They are so obsessed with being accepted by the medics that this split mind still exists. They want so badly to be a recognized physician, but in reality, they have to acknowledge that they are chiropractors.

I Never Wanted to Be a Medic

One day, after I entered practice, I used my National College expertise. I medically diagnosed a patient with bursitis of the glenohumeral cavity. I started to line up one of those half-baked remedies to take the place of cortisone that the medics would have prescribed for bursitis. The patient interrupted me and said, "Norm, quit the bullshit. I came here for an adjustment. If I wanted a medical diagnosis, I would have gone to my medic." That confrontation sobered me, and from that time on, I quit trying to make a silk purse out of a sow's ear. I began adjusting people because that is what they want. If they desire medical stuff, there is a medic around the corner, and if they choose holistic care, there is one of those on the next one. Patients know what they want; it is the chiropractors who are confused. Once I concentrated on adjusting the hips and spine, people started coming in, and they have never stopped. My philosophy as a chiropractor is giving patients a proper adjustment at a fee they can afford, which has made all the difference in the success of my practice.

Robert Frost's poem "The Road Not Taken" is a favorite of mine.

> Two roads diverged in a yellow wood,
> And sorry I could not travel both
> And be one traveler, long I stood
> And looked down one as far as I could

To where it bent in the undergrowth;

Then took the other, as just as fair,
And having perhaps the better claim,
Because it was grassy and wanted wear;
Though as for that, the passing there
Had worn them really about the same,

And both that morning equally lay
In leaves no step had trodden black.
Oh, I kept the first for another day!
Yet knowing how way leads on to way,
I doubted if I should ever come back.
I shall be telling this with a sigh
Somewhere ages and ages hence:
Two roads diverged in a wood, and I—
I took the one less traveled by,
And that has made all the difference.

It implies that when there are two choices, it is not always possible to do both at the same time. A decision must be made; that decision is vital to the outcome and can make all the difference. This poem parallels the chiropractic profession, in that it continues to insist on trying to go down both roads at the same time, never making a choice and sticking with it.

If chiropractors are to continue to exist, they all should learn how to give a proper adjustment, and the goal of the chiropractic profession should become that of adjusting 95 percent of the population. I ask why the profession wants to persist in this dichotomy, this schism. The answer can only be for the chiropractic hierarchy's aggrandizement. It is not practical, it is not helping the profession, and it is not helping the public, which is chiropractic's entire reason for existence.

CHAPTER 9

History Tells Us if We Listen

Historians state that Winston Churchill claimed that World War II would not have needed to take place. When Hitler invaded the Rhineland in the spring of 1936, violating the terms of the agreement that ended World War I, Britain and the allies could have confronted Hitler immediately, thus precipitating his fall from power. Instead, they hesitated. They possessed the military capacity and they had the strength, but what they lacked was the courage and the will to act. They chose the path of appeasement, and much suffering followed. Eighty million people died because of Hitler being allowed to gain power.

Eighty years later, people are still suffering throughout the world. Not in as gruesome a scenario as the gas chambers of Hitler's doing but there is another group, who, like the allies in 1936, have the strength and ability to help the sick and suffering of the world. It is the chiropractic profession, with education in their head and talent and expertise in their hands, which could be helping the planet. Everyone can feel better, act better, and cooperate more if their hips are aligned, the sacrum is level, and the spine straight. But no, chiropractors do not open their doors to let the people in and give them the adjustment they are seeking. The chiropractors are like the allies in trying to appease Hitler. The profession spends their time and money trying to appease the medics, and guess what, the medical profession does not give a darn about the chiropractic profession. The poor profession makes a fool of themselves sucking up to the medics and other agencies. They say, "Hey! Don't leave me out. I, too, am a physician" like the allies who let millions of people be slaughtered during World War II by trying to appease their adversaries.

The chiropractic profession is letting millions in the United States alone go to bed in terrible pain and suffering. Much of that could be alleviated and controlled if people had access to affordable chiropractic care. Why can we not learn from history? Chiropractors have been trying to appease the medics for the last eighty to ninety years, but where has it gotten the profession?

One-Upping the Medics

Almost everyone in existence could use chiropractic care, but because of the multiple personalities the profession possesses, it loves to spend most of its time taking care of medical failures. Because the profession wants to be an "I, too, am a physician," they love to one-up the medic. Patients have made the rounds; they have seen two or three family doctors, two or three specialists, been to Mayo's or the Cleveland Clinic. No one has been able to solve their problem, and as a last resort, they get to a chiropractor. Chiropractors love to get their hands on these chronic cases. They promise these patients three to six months of care, giving the patient tremendous hope. They set up a treatment program that requires the patient to come to the office every day or every other day. This procedure requires a big chunk of time on the part of the patient. It also extracts a bunch of money, sometimes bleeding the patient of their assets, but all this attention gives them hope.

Earlier we said that 80 percent of patients that use chiropractic would get good results, and so it is with these chronic cases. The percentage of "chronics" that get better is very high, high enough that the chiropractor gets giddy when they can help a patient that the medics couldn't. That makes their day. It is impressive that so many chronics do have success. Living without pain is fantastic, and often when we do not have pain, we take it for granted. Sadly, success with these chronic patients does not turn into a massive boon for the chiropractor's practice. Getting rid of a long-standing debilitating problem should be exciting for the patient. Still, most of the time, the patient is relatively blasé about what the chiropractor has accomplished for them.

The primary reason the patient is not that ecstatic is because of the time it took to go to the office so frequently and the high cost, which often comes out of their pocket. Yes, they received fantastic results, but the chiropractors asked so much out of them for their time and money. Because the patient was exhausted from the pain they had endured for so long and the chiropractor asked for more, it became bittersweet. "I love you, chiropractor, but I have had enough of you." A high percentage of the time, the chiropractor will not get a referral from the patient to whom they have just given a new lease on life. It's such a sad scenario and is one of the reasons the profession only sees 5 percent of the public, even with such tremendous results. The patient does not refer their friends and relatives by saying, "Hey, you have to go see this great chiropractor of mine."

While my profession spends all its time on a few chronic cases, the other 95 percent of the population conforms to the whims of our present health-care system. The prescribing of drugs and more drugs that they call healthcare. Chiropractors need to get their heads out of the sand and listen to the polls and the public who say they would love to get an adjustment if the chiropractors would let them. Chiropractors, please remove the barricades, open your doors, let in the people!

Bad Business

The chiropractic profession has "acres of diamonds" (a phrase made famous in a speech by Russell Conwell) in their backyard. Everyone needs an adjustment at one time or another. Regrettably, for the last eighty years, the profession has worn dark glasses and blinders. They sit in their empty offices bemoaning, *Why oh why, don't new patients flock through our door when we get such positive results with our patients?* They pound their chests and say we are as good as the medics—we get people better faster and quicker than they do! However, these patients who got well may not be as excited as the chiropractor when they were required to go to the chiropractor's office every day for six months.

Chiropractors typically do get excellent and fast results, and they do have a good reason to beat their chests. Because chiropractors do not release the patient who received great results after two or three weeks of treatment, the patient becomes turned off even though a miracle did occur. Since chiropractors keep patients coming after they are feeling better, they become burned out. They are not eager to encourage their family or friends to become mired in a similar situation. This type of patient management turns a positive experience into the reason chiropractors are not flooded with new patients and why the profession is seeing only 5 percent of the population.

The chiropractic profession does a great job of helping people. As soon as they help, they turn around and shoot themselves in the foot by not releasing the excited patient when they need to be released. However, before they shoot their foot, they pull another bone-headed stunt. By telling the patient before their initial treatment, "I can help you, but before I do, I want you to pay me for six months care upfront. I will discount the amount, and you will be paying less in the long run than if you were paying per visit." In other words, the chiropractor is, in effect, borrowing money from the patient. How many times have you been told never to cosign a note? How many times have you been told not to loan money when there is no guarantee that you will get it back? The chronic patient says, "Doc, I'll pay you anything you ask to help me," which is why the chiropractor loves the chronic patient. The problem arises when they apply this business plan to all patients, not just the chronics.

A contract to borrow money from patients is a poor business model, and it has been a dreadful business procedure in the profession for years. All the chiropractic magazines and publications ask over and over why we cannot see more patients. At the same time, they promote this business model as acceptable, asking the patient to pay upfront for services before they are rendered.

Are you beginning to see why our profession sees such a small percentage of the population? It's partially because of its practice-management system. It takes one step forward then one step back. The profession exists because it gets results. Until it can see the diamonds in their backyard, I guess there is not a lot of hope for you to receive superb adjustments and improved health.

Meanwhile

While we let the chiropractors feel sorry for themselves and bemoan their plight, I will show you something that may improve your overall structure. It may keep you away from backaches that might arise from wearing improper shoes. Like the shower exercise, it won't cost a dime.

PROPER SHOES

1. Wrong shoe patterns will create structural problems.
2. To find your foot style, wet your foot, place it on paper, use scissors to cut out your foot pattern.

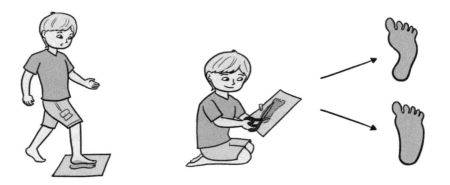

3. Take your paper pattern along when purchasing your next pair of shoes.
4. Turn the shoe over, place foot pattern over the sole of the shoe. Does it match the bottom of the shoe's sole? If yes, it is a buy. If no, forget it.

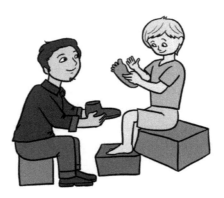

CHAPTER 10

Archaic Habits

Chiropractic was founded in 1895 and is still clinging to its past. It is the twenty-first century, they should move on, but they cannot get away from their old-fashioned ways mired in the nineteenth century. Even in the days of the Old Testament, when one was in business, it had to be a reciprocal act—giving and taking, exchanging and trading. The chiropractic profession has not learned how to reciprocate with their patients. Years ago, the medical profession assaulted and attacked chiropractors and nearly got rid of them. At that time, the profession circled its wagons to fend off and protect itself from attack and took what it could get, which is understandable. Jim Parker, a chiropractor whom we will discuss later, helped save the profession from extinction by devising a practice program chiropractors could use when managing their patients.

It consisted of borrowing money from patients. He observed that there are a lot of chronically ill people who will pay anything to feel better. Dr. Jim's idea was to ask desperate patients for the entire fee upfront to solve their problems. It was remarkable how many chronic patients would pay the whole cost in advance of any care given. It worked well enough with his patients that he started seminars for chiropractors to teach them how to be financially successful using this system. Many chiropractors employed his program, and the profession was able to survive.

It was a stopgap measure and was necessary at the time. It helped the chiropractors financially but was not a program that would allow chiropractors to help and serve the masses. It was not a reciprocal program; it was a one-directional business transaction. The chiropractor received a considerable bonus upfront. One half of the fee that the patient would have paid on a per-visit basis had it not been discounted for the advance-payment cost. In the next several months, the patient received great results, moderate results, or no results.

When you pay the chiropractor the 50 percent discounted $3,000 upfront for your condition, to the patient, it sounds like a substantial promise or guarantees that they will get results. However, when you walk out of the chiropractor's office, unlike the shopkeeper that gives you a sack full of goodies, you leave with nothing. The spinal adjustment that you receive is intangible, and there is no guarantee that it will do a bit of good. If the chiropractor does not produce good results, what sort of taste will be in the mouth of the patient? They shelled out $1,500, thinking that a miracle was going to be performed, but it did not happen? Yikes! That is hard to swallow. Oh, I know my fellow chiropractors will say, "Hey, the medics do it all of the time, and it's true, they do."

We see it almost every day. A patient came in yesterday with back pain, from the hip replacement she had a year ago, to be resolved. She had just come from the doctor who replaced it. After reexamining the hip, he said, "Laura, the hip we replaced is fine. It is in great shape. Your problem is in your back." She said to herself, "Yeah, sure!" Once they have replaced the hip or knee, they dismiss you. Whether it helped or not, the medics can get by with not having to follow up a botched job. However, because the medical doctors can skate and do not have to follow through, the chiropractors ask why can't we slide as well.

The reason the medics get by with it is that they take insurance money, so no one gives a darn if things do not go right. The doctor and surgery center got paid, and there is always a pain clinic if you are not better. However, with chiropractic, the patient, in many instances, is putting up their own money, not the insurance company. When the "miracle," promised for $3000, is not performed, this stops any reciprocity that chiropractors rely on to stay in practice. The medics do not need to satisfy their patients to have a full office; they are the only game in town. For chiropractors to help the suffering masses, they need satisfied patients to reciprocate and send in their friends and relatives. Unfortunately, this does not happen when the patient feels they have been conned. Chiropractors have to understand the medic doesn't need the patient satisfied because they have no competition; they have a 1:1,200 patient-population ratio. The medics do not have to ask the patient for a loan; they call the insurance company for their vast fees.

Conning the patient is much the same problem of loaning money or signing a note for someone. When a loan is not repaid because the results were not satisfactory, hard feelings develop and issues occur. The situation is regrettable because there is so much good in chiropractic, and the profession shouldn't be sitting on the sideline. It is time for the profession to shed its old ways and agree to help all people in this new millennium.

CHAPTER 11

Assuming the Burden

When doctoral programs were set up in the early 1900s, they were designed so that doctors would shoulder the responsibility for pursuing the best course of care for the patient. Technically, that is still the premise of doctoring today. Oaths that doctors take state that a patient's welfare or well-being is foremost. When the medics attacked and the chiropractors circled their wagons to ward off the establishment in the 1930s and 1940s, the Parker format was used to accomplish this feat. In the process of using his procedure, they reversed the burden of responsibility and placed it on the patient. To this day, the chiropractic profession practices this business model. Presently, there are over sixty practice-building companies in the country that teach chiropractic graduates how to use a procedure that will make them a small fortune. Most of their methods are a take-off of the Parker prototype. It shows how to set up the money trap (e.g., forty visits in six months, how to sell the patient on extensive care and how to get new patients).

Since the 1940's, the profession has not changed its patient-management format. They will not let the patient be a reciprocal part of their practice. You, the patient, needs to be included. That is why I previously explained how you could check your hips. Patients want a chiropractor to have an office that is alive and vibrant. They want it to be a respite, a home away from home, a place to go for help any time they need it. That is what reciprocity is all about, an equal give-and-take system with fees that are affordable for the entire family. Most chiropractors, if they are truthful, could not afford to go to themselves because they charge too much. Offices should operate on a cash basis to alleviate the fraud and dishonesty that go along with insurance and governmental programs. When the chiropractor equally shares the burden with the patient, everyone has a successful experience.

The Forest

It is too bad that the administrators of the profession cannot see the forest for the trees. They have such a narrow vision, either acceptance by the government and insurance industry or nothing. If the profession were free to adjust all the spines in the world, what a difference that would make in health care and society. Chiropractic has proven itself beyond any doubt. It gets results, period. There is scientific proof in journals. It just isn't mainstream and will never be as long as the medics are in control.

Patients love to testify that after getting adjusted, they can get up and go to work, which was impossible before the adjustments. Testimonials are the chiropractor's main "scientific proof." Regrettably, as you know, testimonials are not counted as science. Therefore, chiropractors cannot use testimonials of successful resolutions for patients to obtain anything from governmental, insurance, or scientific entities. They say you cannot prove your testimonials, so you do not get to play with us. And we are not going to share our toys (i.e. money) with you.

After one-hundred-plus years of getting nowhere, it is time for the chiropractic hierarchy to teach students how to give a specific physical adjustment and send them out to heal the world. Give people, communities, and patients what they want, which is specific spinal and hip adjustments at affordable fees that make them feel better. They do not want a bunch of other modalities that pad the bill. If the profession would use some good old common horse sense, we could be seeing 95 percent of the population. Many people are now shut out or cannot afford to go to a chiropractor.

Way Off Base

New patients are the lifeblood of any profession. The average chiropractor sees five new patients per week but has the potential to see many more. Unfortunately, chiropractors block their doors with high fees. It becomes imperative for them to attend seminars to learn how to entrap new patients who come to them each week. Many times, patients cannot get started with a chiropractor unless they pay a fee of four hundred dollars to consult with the doctor and have X-rays taken. That initial fee blocks the door for many people, no matter how wonderful the results.

Notwithstanding is the substantial cost of $1,500–$4,000 to solve the case. The profession cannot see the forest. They focus on taking care of one tree and squeezing all the sap out of it that they can when there are thousands of other trees that they could care for as well. Collecting a little sap out of each tree in the forest would benefit everyone. Maybe with your help and my encouragement, the hierarchy will take a second look, see the forest, and become a custodian for the masses who would love an adjustment.

CHAPTER 12

Common Sense

The chiropractic philosophy is a common-sense approach to health. Chiropractic is not rocket science. It is the detection of structural misalignment in the spine and pelvis and the resetting of that malposition. *It is as simple as that!* If chiropractors would just allow the multitudes of people to come to them, every chiropractor's office door would be swinging off its hinges.

Being Liked

In college, I wanted to date a girl I thought I really liked, and eventually, I did have two or three dates with her. However, I found out that if she got what she thought was a better date, I got stood up. This is what the chiropractic profession is doing to you. You are getting stood up. Only the people that can pay the hefty fee or have a good insurance plan are accepted.

The profession spends its time figuring out how to be scientific to receive insurance and grant money. The drive for acceptance at present is focusing on lobbying legislators to allow them to write script. How will our writing scripts help you? Will it make you more appreciative of the profession because they can give you a bottle of pills to take home? Not really, but it will cover up a lot of shortcomings. Since chiropractors charge such outlandish fees if the patient is not better in several visits, they would be able to give the patient drugs to cover up the pain. It might make the patient admire the chiropractor in the short term, but the problem will still exist when the drug wears off. Disastrously, today's chiropractor is not as proficient in adjusting as the old-time chiropractors were. Today, many use machines, adjusting guns, or computerized adjusting tools in place of manual adjusting.

Have you noticed when you go to your medical doctor, they never physically examine you anymore? They send you for tests, and these tests tell them what is wrong with you. It is much the same with modern chiropractors; they do not want to touch you either. In the old days, we had to practice adjusting over and over until we became proficient. We were taught to palpate the spine and hips and use the expertise in our hands to correct subluxations. Today computer adjusting is much easier than developing competency. There is less need to place hands on the patient because the machine does the adjusting for you. However, what happens when these adjusting machines fail? Will the modern chiropractor then cover up the patient's problem by writing a script for painkillers?

If chiropractors were allowed to write script today, I would estimate 50 percent of the younger ones would jump on the idea. Chiropractic is physical work, and it's hard to get off your duff and adjust a three-hundred-pound patient with a hip problem. How much easier would it be to sit across the desk and write a script for pain pills? If chiropractors do get script privileges, that would be like hitting the lottery for them. You would be stood up again. No one is going to like the profession any better because you could get a script from them. No, what you want are chiropractors who have common sense and make themselves available to adjust you.

CHAPTER 13

Clouded Vision

Today's modern chiropractor says if we, as a profession, are ever to be accepted, we have to write script. Over 39 million people are killed, injured, given unnecessary treatments or drugs, or are infected by medical doctors each year.[4] "The most stunning statistic, however, is that the total number of deaths caused by conventional medicine is an astounding 783,936 per year. It is now evident that the American medical system is the leading cause of death and injury in the US."[5] How sad that our profession's goal and vision is to assist the medical profession in creating more drug dependency. My profession is selfish. It is called me-ism and is all about me. They want their vocation to be acceptable, but to whom? The profession is willing to add more drug statistics to the 2.2 million adverse reactions and 128,000 deaths from properly prescribed and administered medications each year. This death rate is "nearly five times the number of people killed by overdosing on prescription painkillers and heroin."[6] Just to become accepted by insurance companies and governmental agencies? Let me ask you, in your everyday life with your family and acquaintances, how many people who only think about themselves do you like? Self-centered people are not very likable, and any profession can also be unlikable if they only think of themselves.

---

[4] Death By Medicine by Gary Null, PhD et al. http://www.webdc.com/pdfs/death-bymedicine.pdf

[5] ibid

[6] Death By Prescription By Michael O. Schroeder, 9/27/16. US News and World Report. https://health.usnews.com/health-news/patient-advice/articles/2016-09-27/the-danger-in-taking-prescribed-medications

After all these years in practice, I have found that patients want an *alternative*. They want an *adjustment*. They do not wish to take more pills. Unfortunately, the chiropractic profession is not listening to you. Chiropractic is for the public, not the chiropractor, a person who has the skill to adjust can see hundreds and hundreds of patients and help them. I would bet the back forty that if I would not set a fee on my adjustment but put a box by the door for donations and adjust as many people as I could day after day, I would be a very wealthy person. I would have riches of all kinds—spiritual, friendships, and monetarily. Today the public is taking a backseat to good health care that chiropractors could offer them because the chiropractic profession is wrapped up in itself wanting to be *the* doctor. Therefore, typically, the only way you can get chiropractic care today is to have an excellent insurance policy or $1,500-$4,000 of cash handy. Again, is chiropractic for the public or the chiropractor?

Folks say to me, "Oh, Norm, you are so archaic! This is the future. One of these days, it will be all machines, computers, and paperless. Tax money will go into the system, and all you will have to do is tap your pad. Information will be transferred directly into your account, and bingo, you will have your fee. You will get your money no matter how you treat your patient. It will make no difference whether you are kind or not." They say, "Get with it, Norm. The future is technology, the sciences, new and exciting medicines, and we want our profession to be on board. We cannot be left out."

Change

Progressives in the hierarchy of the chiropractic profession want us to adapt to changes in science, technology, and medicine and want us to become scientific. If the profession gravitates to these scientific changes, will these changes help you? The answer is a resounding no! No, the changes will not help you one iota!

There is a marvelous book titled *Business Secrets from the Bible* by Rabbi Daniel Lapin. In the chapter titled "Secret #24: The More That Things Change, The More We Must Depend Upon Those Things That

Never Change,"[7] he states that life primarily consists of six different compartments: science, technology, medicine, man, nature, and God. He spends eleven pages discussing how science, technology, and medicine are always changing, but God, nature, and man never change. He goes on to say, change is necessary, but to cope with the constant flux of change, you need the pillars of God, nature, and man for guidance going forward.

For centuries, we worshipped God. Today, liberalism teaches that God is mythical and does not exist, and they are doing everything to see that God is removed from our lives and is cast aside.

This allows us to worship at the altar of technology, science, and drugs. One of the reasons we spend so much time studying and bowing down to these three is because technology is exciting. Look at how everyone spends time with computers, texting, and Facebook. Medicine and all the new physiologically altering drugs that are on the market are almost overwhelming. I am sure that is why churches are emptying with people no longer attending. There is very little time for God anymore.

There are times when change is necessary; we all know this to be true. However, there are also times when things should never ever change! Chiropractic is one of those. Chiropractic is a combination of God, nature, and man; it is not science. The body has not changed for eons of time unless you want to believe in evolution, which says we evolved from four-legged beings to monkeys and then into humans. God created man to stand upright. We are the only living being that stands upright, eats with a knife and fork, and drinks out of a glass. In the process of standing upright, we have many moving components, along with coordination to allow us to keep our balance and the ability to do many things that animals cannot do.

In performing all these remarkable feats, we still can keep our joints in their proper place. When the vertebra of the body goes out of place, it is called a subluxation. The body will then do all within its power to put it back in its proper position. When the body cannot reposition itself, it will do everything it can to solidify that joint. In doing so,

[7] Business Secrets from the Bible—Spiritual Success Strategies for Financial Abundance by Rabbi Daniel Lapin. Published by John Wiley & Sons, 2014

it will not be too mobile and will create other issues. When the body hardens a hypermobile joint, this is called arthritis, which is nothing more than callus formation. The callus is laid down to cement the bone from being too floppy and mobile, creating more damage. That is why it is imperative to keep the hips level. By having a chiropractor level the sacral base and align the spine, callus formation or arthritis will not have a chance to build. The body tries everything it can to readjust the misaligned parts and close the structural gap that trauma or repetitive overuse produces. Occasionally, this fails, and the chiropractor steps in to help. The chiropractor finds a vertebra located at point B that needs to be in its proper position at point A. Once the misalignment is found, the chiropractor sets it in motion so it can return to point A. The innate intelligence of the body begins to reposition it to take the pressure off any nerve involved. Organization and normal functions are returned to the structure or organ that was affected. The analysis of the spine and correction of a subluxated vertebra has not changed since chiropractic was founded. Incidentally, this would have been the same in the time of Jesus Christ because the body has not changed and nature has not changed.

If nothing has changed in the human body since the time of Christ and the job of the chiropractor has not changed, why then do we need to bring science into the format of chiropractic education? Chiropractic is the combination of nature and man, two things that never change, and it relies on God's power to allow the body to heal when the interference is out of the way.

So far, science for chiropractic has not validated a hypothesis or observation that chiropractic works. Experimentation on living upright human beings cannot be performed as it can on four-legged animals. Chiropractic is like nature and God—it works! How many times have you been in awe and asked yourself, "How does nature know when to have the buds come out in the spring?" I am sure scientists have their theories, but do you or I know them? No, but the buds come out every spring. Just the same, maybe chiropractic should not have been classified as a science—chiropractic being aligned with the unchanging but necessary fundamental aspects we discussed. How important it is to humanity that we get away from the obsession of belonging to the ever-changing world of technology, science, and medicine. When this occurs, good things will happen for all humankind.

If we take one part sodium and one part chloride and mix them, it produces table salt. This process can be duplicated over and over, and each time, the combination provides salt. It can be validated as the process will produce the same result every time. This is science, the observation of a concept or method that will work time and time again. In chiropractic, doctor A can adjust patient B's fourth dorsal vertebrae with a posterior to anterior move and get a great result. Doctor C can adjust patient B's fourth dorsal vertebrae with a posterior to anterior, and the results may be different or nonexistent. This issue of duplication has kept chiropractic out of the realm of science. Yes, we can duplicate adjusting the same vertebra, manifesting the same problem, but because of the human factor, the outcome may differ. For example, doctor C maybe a foot shorter than doctor A. Therefore, the line of the drive of the two doctors will be different. This will cause the correction of the vertebra to vary between the two doctors, thus producing a different outcome. However, in science, one part sodium and one part chloride equal salt every time.

The irony of this is that the duplication of research procedures for medicine or drugs can be formulated time and time again in the laboratory; therefore, it is science. However, the result of that formula does not always produce the same results due to physiological differences in patients. In reality, medicine's ability to get results is not 100 percent. It would be interesting to see the actual rate of help medicines do produce when duplicated in different patients with the same condition. I will almost guarantee the rate is not very high. I base this on my years of experience seeing patients and hearing comments on their success rate.

It is also my opinion that chiropractors should quit lamenting the fact that we are not scientific. When it comes down to it, medics passing out pills do not get any better results than we chiropractors for many maladies. When a tablet goes into the body, most of the time, it is a shot in the dark as to whether it will help. Also, how often do patients go back to the doctor to say the medication didn't help? What percent say,

"Hey, Doc, that prescription helped. It did the trick"? I am convinced that there is very little follow-up as to what pill worked and which did not and, more importantly, why it did or did not.

Chiropractors need to recognize that science is not all it claims because it is always changing. A vertebra out of place today will be out of place tomorrow unless corrected by the body or set in motion by a chiropractor. We need to realize that we have a much-needed service. It was needed yesterday, it is needed today, and it will be needed tomorrow throughout the entire world. Wow! Man and nature do not change; gravity does not change. Humans, with all our mobility and activities, will be susceptible to hip misalignment and vertebra being out of place. We will need a chiropractor to help get back on track whether science is involved or not. The chiropractic profession believes we need to be scientific to prove ourselves. Patients do not care if we are; they want an effective adjustment and do not want us to change.

CHAPTER 14

Givers and Takers

The chiropractic profession is still living and existing in the protection mode of the nineteenth and twentieth centuries. We are still working hard to please the scientific world, the same world that tried to eliminate the entire profession. Chiropractic has always taken the backseat and gets excited to receive table scraps when the medics set up front and get all the excellent insurance pickings. They live high off of the hog with the pork chops, tenderloins, and ham the insurance companies hand out. John Mortimer wrote a series of stories about Rumpole, a lawyer in the Old Bailey Court of London. Rumpole refers to his wife as "she who must be obeyed." It is a delightful series, and Rumpole is a funny character who quotes Shakespeare. There is much tragedy in Shakespeare's work, but I cannot help but compare Rumpole's obeying and Shakespeare's tragedies to the chiropractic profession. We are so pleased to bow to "they (science and medicine) who must be obeyed." We grin, jump up and down, shout, sing, and are happy scavenging the leftovers and tidbits the medics throw our way. This leads to the tragedy that we only see 5 percent of the population, and the remainder has no concept of or access to chiropractic. It is a tragedy that the hierarchy of our profession wants us to mimic the medics—these same medics who imposed rules and regulations to satisfy insurance companies, governmental, and other institutional entities. All of whom are more focused on their financial well-being than on patient's health and welfare.

The medics can get by with treating people deplorably because they can tap into the insurance industry that was put into place for them. The insurance companies and medics are a marriage. The chiropractic profession wants to be a live-in, set at the same table, cut into all that delicious pork that the medical insurance couple gets to dine on every day. It is never going to happen; the medical/insurance couple does not want a boarder. However, what the household throws in the garbage satisfies the chiropractic profession.

Here is the bittersweet truth: you who need chiropractic care so badly will have to keep suffering, while the insurance industry gives scraps to the chiropractors.

1.) Insurance companies allow chiropractors a set number of visits per diagnosed case. It may vary with the diagnosis, but say the average is ten.

2.) The insurance company will pay up to one hundred dollars per visit.

3.) The chiropractor will program the patient's care around these ten visits.

4.) Once that set number is exhausted, the chiropractor has to reexamine the patient, change the diagnosis, and start over with another diagnosis. This procedure will go on until the patient tires of trips to the chiropractor, the patient feels better and stops on his own, or the insurance company ceases to pay.

5.) The chiropractor will usually get the patient to retain at least twenty visits.

6.) The chiropractor may average twenty-five patient visits per day.

7.) At one hundred dollars per patient times twenty-five visits, this would equal $2,500 a day income.

8.) If the chiropractor is in the office from nine to five, five days a week, $2,500 times five equals $12,500 per week.

9.) If the chiropractor practices fifty weeks a year, fifty times 12,500 per week equals $725,000 per year income.

10.) This is why, when I talk to my fellow chiropractors about lowering the cost of an adjustment to allow patients to flow into their office, they scoff at me.

11.) Chiropractic is possibly one of the most lucrative fields in existence because of low overhead.

12.) The rate $725,000 per year for seeing very few patients is nothing at which to sneeze. You can see why chiropractors are happy to take home the bacon—oops, I mean scraps! They complain about not seeing more people and not receiving more recognition. But no way are they going to take less money to see more people. It is not going to happen, period.

Tragedy

I have kept a diary of my daily activities and events in my office since 1966. One of these recordings is what I call a tragic story. It's not like losing a loved one, but to me, it is a tragedy because of what might have been.

Jane, a seventy-four-year-old widow, decided to join an exercise class at the local gym. Most instructors at a gym are young, slender, and lean. Jane tried to keep up with them, and you can guess what happened. She began to have hip pain and leg discomfort at first, and then severe pain in both areas developed so that sleeping and sitting were unbearable. Off she went to the medic for X-rays, therapy, and pills. After three weeks of no sleep or relief, she was referred to me by our neighbor. I adjusted her two days in a row, and the second adjustment lessened the pain 80 percent. Wow, was she excited! After two days of relief, her kids came from out of town to visit. They took her around town, and it was just too much activity. The adjustment had not set up enough for all this activity, and the severe pain returned. She told her family she wanted to go to the chiropractor, and they would not hear of that. "You are going to the hospital where you will get good care, and you are not going back to that chiropractor"—in other words, "that quack." They were adamant that she would go back to the medics and follow through with their "good care."

She listened to her kids and followed the medical doctor's orders. For the next three months, she was in constant moderate to severe pain. Also, she developed stomach ulcers from all the medication. Her lifestyle was interrupted for five months. Eventually, she sneaked into our office for two more adjustments, and all her pain disappeared. Granted this was after three months of therapy, but when we first adjusted her, she got immediate relief. Would the comfort have continued after the first two adjustments? I believe she would have needed five or six adjustments and would have been fine in two or three weeks instead of suffering for five or six months.

Yes, it is tragic and unfortunate that chiropractic is not seeing 95 percent of the population. If we were, we would not have to worry about being accepted; we would be! Under these circumstances, Jane's kids would not have stuck their noses in with their tainted view. Since I was a "quack," their decision made their mother suffer and go through three additional months of suffering needlessly. However, I cannot fault them. I do blame the chiropractic profession for allowing practitioners to take scraps for selfish reasons.

How many people, like Jane, suffer needlessly because we sit idly by waiting to be accepted scientifically? If we were accepted, Jane's kids would not have called me a quack and would have let me take care of her. If we as a profession are seeing the mass of the population and getting results, do you think the public would give a hoot if we are scientific? No way! If we get results and people can afford to come to us, I will guarantee the world will be at the chiropractor's doorstep. We need to be adjusting all of God's children, and it is possible. The profession needs to accept the fact that the body does not change, that we are a part of God and nature, and that that never changed. We are not in the science, medicine, and technology group that is always evolving. Spinal subluxations have plagued man since he has existed. Most of the time, the body will correct subluxations on its own, but there are times when it needs help. Once the profession sets out to make this their mission, then the world will begin to feel better.

Once our profession sees that we can make the most significant impact in changing the world's health by adjusting the spine, we will be accepted. There is a second problem that chiropractors need to resolve. Many of today's chiropractors are takers and not givers. A law of life that has been around forever is that we must give before we receive. Chiropractors, to protect their gains when they were being persecuted so severely, went into the mode of giving once they got. Unfortunately, they have not given up their old business model. It has been very destructive for the growth of the profession.

Quit Loaning Money

You, the public, need to stop loaning chiropractors money to take care of you. It is not a good business policy for either you or the chiropractor. When you lend the chiropractor money upfront, 90 percent of the time, you will never need all the care they recommend. The chiropractor gets a nice nest egg upfront and possibly hopes you will never collect on all those visits. Chiropractors have been borrowing money from their patients for the last seventy years. They get you to loan them $2,000 to take care of your case by paying for your care upfront. They will want you to come into the office three times per week for six months. Unfortunately, this allows the chiropractor to become enslaved to the patient. They have to make you happy for six months. That becomes a problem if they have to entertain you for six months if you have gotten better in three or four visits. At this point, you have to be convinced to return for the remaining visits. Many chiropractors have gyms, exercise equipment, massage, etc. to keep you interested and happy during this remaining time.

Today's chiropractors are takers. They accept your "loan" based on a false premise that you need all that care when in reality, there is no guarantee that you will get well. The assumption is that when the patient forks over that big loan to the chiropractor, they will get well, and it is at that point, the chiropractor becomes enslaved to you. What happens if you do not get well?

For the profession to grow and thrive, it has first to learn how to give. Giving and serving humanity is what chiropractors can do better than any other profession on earth. But it has to reverse its way of thinking from waiting to give until they receive. The law of nature is straightforward; we reap what we sow—ask any farmer.

Reformation of the profession is badly needed to change old policies that were installed to protect chiropractors in the early years. The medical profession was vehement about destroying and getting rid of "quacks, cultists, and charlatans" once and for all. We now know the medics were wrong! There is a definite need for the structural and functional components of the body to be respected because it plays a significant role in the health-care equation. It has proven itself time and time again. Yet the medical profession still has the power to dominate the licensing laws as to how chiropractors can present themselves to the public. These laws that were developed to control yesterday's chiropractors are still on the books today. The US Constitution states that changes to the constitution have to be mandated by the voice of the people, not by the courts. Until the chiropractic profession and the public have the initiative and courage to stand up and tell the medical court to go to hell, chiropractors will continue to see only a few patients. The chiropractic closed shops will continue to exist, and many of you will be denied the right to a good adjustment. We should all be raging mad at this!

Until the chiropractors can see a way to get all people a proper adjustment, I have a little trick for you. It doesn't cost a dime but will make you feel better if you do it consistently until you can get an adjustment.

YELLOW ONIONS AND THE TUMMY

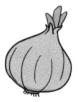

"It was my grandmother's belief and it is also mine, eating a small yellow (raw) onion daily will keep the stomach fine."

"Most all gastritis and ulcer patients will be helped or cured and not just a few. But it has to be a yellow onion and not a red, white or blue,"

Do not ask why, just do it. It works!

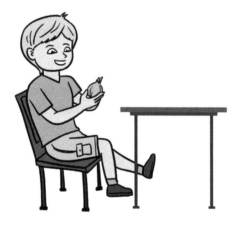

CHAPTER 15

The Reformations of Chiropractic

In the early days, shortly after the discovery of chiropractic, it found itself in hot water with the long arm of the medical profession. Medical doctors were in charge of the health-care field; they were the supreme bosses. It would be over their dead body that an "upstart" profession was going to gain entrance into their domain, their territory, or their club.

In the long run, no matter how hard they tried to beat down these upstarts, hold them to the mat, and bloody their noses, they could not put the chiropractors away. They could not destroy them.

Chiropractic survived because of the truth that it works, even without scientific proof, but at a terrible price. Because the medics could not get rid of us, they determined to control our activities through the legislature, and our survival and destiny would be on their terms.

Due to the medic's decree, chiropractic has dealt with five major issues that continue to plague the growth of the profession. These issues have impeded your opportunity to be checked for structural alignment, allowing you to have a more pain-free life.

These issues consist of (1) how chiropractors are licensed, (2) how a lack of competition for medical doctors affects and stymies chiropractic growth, (3) practice builders in the chiropractic profession, (4) insurance and how it corrupts the health industry, and (5) how medical intrusion has adversely affected the chiropractic curriculum.

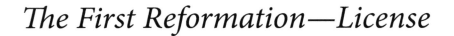

The First Reformation—License

CHAPTER 16

The Right to Bait and Switch

Let me explain how the issue of licensing affects you. For example, let's say you live in Rhode Island. Your chiropractor gives you an incredible adjustment that keeps you functioning well for six months at a time. You like the results, and you encourage your friend in Chicago to seek a chiropractor so they, too, can experience that remarkable relief. When your friend finds a chiropractor and goes to the office, they are instead talked into an acupuncture treatment. Another friend in Des Moines who you encourage to go for an incredible adjustment may wind up with a massage instead. Then you encourage a friend in Dallas to get an adjustment. When they go to the chiropractor, they alternatively receive fifteen physical therapy visits.

Chiropractic has been branded and rightfully so. The brand is that chiropractors adjust the spine. That is what people believe we do, are good at, and what they want when they go to a chiropractor. But the laws in most states are very broad and allow anything that is generally considered holistic to be permitted under the chiropractic practice act. It is interesting that none of the holistic therapies are licensed, only chiropractic. Therefore, the adjusting aspect of chiropractic is the engine that is pulling all these adjunctive therapies along. There is no uniformity in chiropractic offices across the country. If you go to twenty offices, you may get twenty different workups and treatment protocols. We are genuinely branded, but there is no conformity.

If you go to a medical doctor's office, you will be prescribed drugs. At a dental office, you will receive cleaning and tooth repair. At an optometrist's office, your eyes will be checked and fitted with glasses or contacts. Yes, there is uniformity but not at a chiropractor's office. There you may get almost any health-care treatment imaginable. Some of the more common ones are laser therapy, kinesiology, physical therapy, nutritional counseling, vitamin therapy, homeopathy, colonic irrigations, reflexology, hair analysis, and weight reduction. Also, there is massage, Rolfing, facial sculpting procedures, colored lights, and hypnotherapy. The list goes on and on.

Today's state laws that govern and control the practice of chiropractic are very broad. The modern chiropractor is protected and allowed to practice almost anything under the sun. Exceptions are pulling teeth, writing drug prescriptions, performing major surgery, or fitting glasses. Chiropractors can practice nearly any form of alternative medicine they want. Talk about giving someone enough rope to hang themselves; the medics sure knew what they were doing!

Why is this a good deal for the medics and a poor one for you and the chiropractors? By placing all unlicensed therapies under the chiropractic umbrella, they figured out a way to control all the "quacks."

The old saying "Jack of all trades, master of none" seems to apply. If you give a child twenty toys to play with, usually they can't make up their mind and will often become frustrated with so many choices. If they play with one for ten seconds and another for another ten seconds, they will never master the concept of the toy's design. On the other hand, give a child an old box to play with, and they will play with it all afternoon and design many different uses for it. Restricting chiropractors to adjusting the spine, staying in their field, and doing only that one thing they would become expert structural specialists. They could be seeing masses of the population. Can you see that if everyone in the country had an opportunity to have their spines checked, what a threat that would be to the medical profession? Is it any wonder that the medics are happy that the chiropractic profession is so diversified? It keeps them dabbling around in myriads of alternative fields, which causes chiropractors to be as frustrated as a kid with too many toys. The chiropractors are kept out of the medic's hair and on the other side of the watering hole. When the chiropractors are drinking the lousy water across the way, it keeps them from depleting the medic's patient pool for drug therapy.

Chiropractors love to play with these add-on therapies that are not chiropractic but which are allowed because of the broad laws. There are a tremendous number of chiropractors in the country who are first-rate salespeople, who make big, big money. The January 2016 issue of *Dynamic Chiropractic Magazine* had an advertisement of a practice-building company urging chiropractors to take their course and learn how to make an additional $200,000 per year by showing patients how to lose weight. When the chiropractor is spending time teaching you how to lose weight, how much time are they spending adjusting you? That is what you went to the chiropractor for in the first place, right? You did not go to lose weight!

The laws that have been established by states that allow chiropractors to do so many different procedures create an environment for the old bait-and-switch game.

Your friend from Rhode Island was so excited about her adjustment and wanted you to have the same experience. In Chicago, the chiropractor wants you to receive acupuncture, physical therapy, and traction. They want to do laser therapy, and since you are a little overweight, definitely weight reduction. In all, this will take six months of extensive and almost daily visits. You are flabbergasted when you hear the report that all these therapies are needed. Your friend in Rhode Island said probably two or three adjustments would be required, and you would be on your way. These chiropractors will state, "We will give you an adjustment when we deem it necessary. Our thorough exam found you need other therapies to make you 100 percent well again." Because laws are so broad, this allow many chiropractors to become financially successful because they have a lot to sell. With all the gimmicks and therapies chiropractors have to sell, it does not take many patients to make a small fortune. If they can sell the patient on the premise that their life is in danger if they do not go along with the program, that is their goal. It takes only twenty patients a day at two hundred dollars per visit, five days a week to make $1 million a year.

The majority of chiropractors spend time in their lucrative play-grounds protected by liberal laws and set up by our elected legisla-tures, while the mass of the population, the working men and women, are being cheated by not being treated structurally and having to live with ongoing pain and discomfort. They have to rely on medical doc-tors to dish out opioids, steroids, and Celebrex to cover up their pain. Unfortunately, the opioids are causing more problems with side effects. The structural experts, who could be correcting their issues, sit on their hands as they watch a few gullible patients frolic in their therapy rooms.

Licensing laws are put in place to protect the public and to assure quality care for any given professional service that presents itself to the population. Chiropractic laws have not been scrutinized since their inception. They have only been expanded, but unfortunately, not to the benefit of the public for whom they are to serve and protect. In the above example, when the friend in Chicago went to the chiropractor specifically to get an adjustment, she was sold a six-month package of treatment far removed from the adjustment. She wanted an adjustment, not a generic package deal. Typically, when you think of chiropractic, you think of an adjustment, and that is not what she received. Baiting and switching are not right, and laws have been put in place to protect the consumer. In chiropractic, the laws tend to allow the profession to misapply this quality factor. The patient went to the chiropractor with the intent to get what chiropractor's offer, an adjustment. When the chi-ropractor does not do what is expected, they will lose face in the public realm. And chiropractor's wonder, *Why oh why do we only see 5 percent of the population?* Do you suppose the baiting and switching have anything to do with it?

CHAPTER 17

Bullying

Young chiropractic students head to school with the grandiose ideas of giving and serving others. Unfortunately, today, that trip through chiropractic school exposes our young student to many courses that do not pertain to the actual practice of chiropractic. Schools no longer concentrate on how vital the subluxation is or the necessity of correcting that subluxation. Instead, students are instructed on how to fill out forms that will reap a harvest from the insurance company. They are taught that patients need these additional procedures because they are helpful, they work, and they are licensed to perform them. Trust me; I'm a doctor!

The real reason these therapies are performed, whether needed or not, is because chiropractors cannot get paid handsomely for their adjustments. If a chiropractor sends a bill to the insurance company for four different services totaling $300 for a particular visit, the insurance company reviews the claim. When they get through paring down to the necessary treatment, the chiropractor may only get one third of the amount filed. The three hundred-dollar request will be pared down to between eighty and one hundred dollars that the chiropractor will receive for that visit. This is why chiropractors need to perform many therapies. They need to utilize numerous entities to receive one hundred dollars per visit. Chiropractors have to know how to work the system to stay in business and to determine what level of financial success they will ultimately achieve.

It is an engaging game chiropractors have to play. Insurance companies do not readily recognize subluxations because they believe they are unscientific. Therefore, they do not want to acknowledge the adjustment. A few insurance companies do honor adjustments but not to a significant degree. The irony is that the chiropractic adjustment for the subluxation is what is licensed by law. It is what allows the chiropractor to exist as a health-care provider, yet it is not widely recognized by the government or insurance providers for monetary reimbursement. Ironically, insurance companies will pay quite well for physical therapy, which, in comparison to chiropractic, is approximately one fourth as effective. Irony, you bet! Chiropractic works three or four times better and faster than physical therapy, yet chiropractors cannot get amply reimbursed for the adjustment. They will pay the chiropractor handsomely for administering physical therapy, but chiropractors are not physical therapists. They study very little physical therapy in school. Can you see a problem with this scenario? Chiropractors can get reimbursed for what they are not licensed to do but receive very little for what they are licensed to practice. Do you now see why your Chicago friend became entrapped? If you decide to go to a chiropractor today, there is the potential that you will receive what the chiropractor can get paid for and not necessarily what will be in your best interest.

Health licensing laws historically set by the Government Medical Council (GMC) and the Carnegie Foundation, masterminded by Abner Flexner, was purposely set up to protect the public from dastardly quacks, charlatans, and cultists. The GMC group wanted total control over health care in America. They argued that people needed quality health care that only graduates from their approved schools could provide. Those laws were established in the early 1900s to make medical doctors the king of the hill. It worked exceptionally well. After one hundred years, these laws have not eliminated all their competition. There are many holistic therapies in existence, but it did protect them from competition within their ranks. They do not have to worry about a medic setting up down the street and bleeding off their patients. There are only a specified number allowed to practice and hold a license. If twice as many medical doctors were to graduate, guess what would happen to the cost of health care. The law protects the medical profession from being flooded by ensuring that the law of supply and demand is in operation.

This allows the GMC to say they have had the best quality health care for the last one hundred years. In reality, they allowed chiropractors to be licensed then turned their heads when other holistic therapies were shoved under the umbrella of the chiropractic law. The GMC walked away saying, "We pushed the holistic baggage under the chiropractic tent. Let them take care of them." I am not sure if this was a planned direction or if they were just lucky. Maybe the chiropractic profession was gullible and let this happen because they were desperate to get any crumbs the medics might throw their way. My opinion is the latter. Yes, the laws worked out well for the medical profession, but they can only offer you half the equation, the chemical part. What you have not received is the mechanical half of health care. Health care—all of it, the chemical and mechanical aspects—should be available to the world. When the mechanical half is being denied the public this is a travesty affecting all. It is appalling that students who attend college to learn to be the best chiropractic adjusters they can be are then forced to learn and practice therapies that have nothing to do with and overshadow the power of the chiropractic adjustment.

CHAPTER 18

Change Some Things; Don't Change Others

Licensing laws for the chiropractic profession absolutely must be changed. The responsibility of any licensing body is to protect society. What is the purpose of a driver's license? (1) Yes, it becomes a qualifier that you know how to drive and will not be a hazard on the road. (2) Also, others who come in close contact with you on the way assume that you are a qualified and trained driver and are thus protected. In chiropractic, licensing laws merely attest that the chiropractor has completed his education and testing but are somewhat negligent in protecting the public. Are you taking a big chance when you go to a chiropractor who is practicing fifteen different therapies that he or she is not qualified to deliver? There is no licensing law for these therapies. Most often, what they are using is learned in a downtown hotel throughout a weekend.

The original mandate for chiropractic law was for the chiropractor to safely deliver a high-quality spinal adjustment using what they learned of the normal and abnormal structure of human anatomy. Chiropractic students are without peer as they are thoroughly taught the normal and abnormal spinal anatomy and function. They learn the art of analyzing and adjusting subluxations anywhere in the pelvis and spinal column. The chiropractor's job is to restore and maintain the structural integrity of the spine, thereby releasing the flow of the nervous system. This is what chiropractors were licensed to practice. It was not a license to allow chiropractors to sell and coerce the patient into the myriad of therapies chiropractors force on their patients today. None of these therapies are licensed under chiropractic. Authorities who administer the laws never enforce restrictions; instead, they turn their heads and allow chiropractors to practice whatever they want.

Back to the driver's license scenario. Would it be legal for us to use our driver's license designed for a car to be the same license that we could use to drive an eighteen wheeler? Are you beginning to get the picture? Chiropractors have one license but are allowed to use unlicensed procedures for which they have not been adequately trained or qualified by any testing procedure. As the law stands today, it enables the chiropractors to foist upon you, as a patient, any one of these unlicensed procedures. You went to receive an adjustment; you did not go to pay for things you do not need. Laws that are in place to protect you are not doing their job, and that is a fraud, pure and simple.

In the following chapters, we will discuss how the licensing laws can be changed. We want to protect you from the action of stealing your time and money on therapies and show how a simple change will allow you to see a chiropractor and receive what you need, an adjustment. If the chiropractor insists on wanting to perform other therapies, we will show how it can be done professionally and above board so the chiropractor is not characterized as a fraud and a hustler.

The Second Reformation—The 1:1,200 Ratio

CHAPTER 19

Is There a Doctor Shortage?

The Second Reformation the chiropractic profession has to deal with is a ratio of one medical doctor for every 1,200 people in the country. This 1:1,200 ratio was set up for the medical profession. And they vehemently adhere to it, and they will not waiver in its enforcement. Because of the strict adherence to this ratio, it creates havoc with the chiropractic profession. It is the direct reason the United States has the costliest health-care system in the world. Politicians bluster and haggle about America's health care, Medicare, and national health care. Yet they never come up with any conclusions or solutions, nor will they as long as this ratio of 1:1,200 is allowed to remain in place.

I want all of you to go to your local library and have the librarian pull out the book *The Carnegie Reports*. In the section called "Final Report of the Commission on Medical Education" dated 1932 and on page 120, it states, "Proper medical services can be provided on the basis of one active physician to 1,200 persons in the community."

Yes, ladies and gentlemen, there is a doctor shortage, a genuine doctor shortage. It is a contrived doctor shortage, a manufactured shortage. Yes, they continually lie to us! Do not take my word for it; you can go to the library and see for yourself this hoax that has been foisted upon us. We continuously hear the media and doctors themselves say, "Oh, if we only had more doctors."

In 1905, Andrew Carnegie used much of his amassed fortune from the steel industry to fund a sweeping reformation of education in America. The educational format we now use comes directly from the studies and restructuring that was done because of his influence and the money he contributed to this project.

This restructuring started in kindergarten and continued through elementary, secondary, postsecondary education, and the professions. It ran the whole gamete. When they got to the professional studies, especially the medical field, they felt that they had to have top-quality professionals but limit their numbers. If they controlled the number of medical schools, limited the number of students accepted in those schools along with making it extremely difficult to get through the courses, these steps would stifle the number of medical degrees awarded. By choosing the brightest and sharpest applicants and allowing only one doctor for every 1,200 people in the population, ultimately, we would have the best and highest-quality health care in the world.

Before 1910, each state had several private commercial medical schools training students and granting medical degrees. The committee formed by the Carnegie Institute made up of members of the medical profession and government representatives abolished all commercial schools in every state. At that time, there were no controls over what the schools were teaching, and there was no continuity. Remember, in America in the early days, we had free enterprise because the industrial revolution had taken place. Andrew Carnegie was an example of the free enterprise system and made his fortune with it. If his steel, which at the time had no government controls governing its quality, were not of value, no one would have bought it. The same with commercial medical schools, if the student they put out did not do a good job, no one would go to their doctors. The committee formed by the Carnegie Foundation determined they needed control, so they eradicated all commercial schools in every state. In place of these debunked commercial schools, they set up a government-controlled medical school in each state with a consistent educational format. They permitted each state one, two, three medical schools based on the state's population. For example, Kentucky is a small state and has one medical school. Michigan, a more populated state, has two medical schools, and Illinois has three. Can you guess how many seats are available in each incoming freshman class for these medical schools? You got it! It depends upon the 1:1,200 ratio, which is calculated by the state's population.

Most of the incoming medical classes will have approximately 250 seats available. Not everyone gets into this elite fraternal organization. Medical schools may have five thousand applicants for those 250 seats. In reality, this is not much of a free enterprise system regarding the medical profession. It is a "closed shop" and possibly one of the most effective monopolies or consortiums in America. No one calls it a union, but a union it is. And because it is powerful, as with all influential organizations, they can control the media. Because of their strength, you will continue to hear that there is a doctor shortage, yet they will never tell you they contrived the deficit.

This 1910 reformation of the medical profession took a lot of intestinal fortitude on the part of the medics, government, and finances that Carnegie supplied. It produced a massive change in America's free enterprise system, which continues today. The citizen's right to participate in commerce along with their rights as to the type of health care they want versus what the government wants them to have. Andrew Carnegie would never have had the opportunity to succeed as he did had the government put controls on the production of steel like he helped the government put on health-care providers. The dichotomy of Carnegie's actions is astounding! Carnegie, a free-market capitalist during the industrial revolution creating abundant good for the country and world, used his fortune to start a socialistic/communistic medical structure. It was the beginning of our great country, sliding down the slippery slope of socialism/communism. What a travesty!

Socialism/communism dictates that the government controls everything. The government will tell you what to do and when to do it. Unfortunately, many people want the government to do everything for them. Just look at Bernie Sander's presidential run in 2016. He is a self-avowed communist and has broken the barrier for liberals to admit that they are socialists or communists.

When the government begins to control us, they control all media outlets and tell us what they want us to know. The reality is, if the likes of Bernie Sanders became president, this would happen. How many times recently have you heard on the news that we have a doctor shortage? Now knowing about the 1:1,200 ratio, don't you think the socialist media are duping us? Yes, that is their scheme. Abner Flexner, who put this plan together, admitted it was a monopoly. It has become the most powerful cartel the world has ever known. Once students are accepted into medical school, keep their nose clean, and agree with everything the instructors say, they have it made for life. What other profession is handed a guaranteed clientele upon graduation? The predetermined ratio gives them an automatic 1,200 patients. It is money in the bank that guarantees loans, offers memberships in country clubs, and delivers status in the community. Unless the physician does something morally wrong, they are virtually guaranteed a license for life. Medicine is a monopolistic fraternity. Once the student has paid the price of pledgeship, has been initiated, and subsequently accepted, no fraternal organization in the world will give more protection and privileges than that of a medical doctor.

There is no doctor shortage; it is a planned shortage and an outright lie, which was perhaps America's first and continuous fake news.

CHAPTER 20

Flexnerism, Socialism—One of a Kind

How does this medical socialism relate to chiropractors? How many kids have you heard say, "When I grow up, I want to be a doctor"? How many mothers hope their child becomes a doctor? How many teachers in high school push their best and brightest students into the "elite" of all professions? Medical doctors have one of the most sought-after professions. Every year, there may be several thousand applicants for the 250 freshmen seats available in every medical school in the country. How many of those students will have their dreams shattered by not getting accepted into medical school? Then multiply several thousand by the number of medical schools in America. That is a lot of students left out; do they all have a backup plan? Many of them still want to be doctors, and their mothers still want them to be doctors, so what is next? Can you see where this is going?

Chiropractic schools award doctorates, and the rejected student realizes he can still be a doctor. So they enroll in chiropractic school, and while they won't be a "real" doctor, they can always be a doctor that their mother and teacher wanted. It's better than nothing!

This is how what I call flexnerism, which altered the chiropractic profession. Nothing has been done to remedy it to this day. Chiropractic has become a stopping off place for many applicants that couldn't get into medical school. We do not get all the unaccepted students, but we get enough to mess up our educational system as it now stands. Unaccepted medical applicants flood the chiropractic schools and obstruct our vision and mission.

They enter our field having no knowledge that chiropractic existed until they could not get into medical school. Many have never had an adjustment. They have no experience of structural involvement concerning health care; they accept chiropractic as a last resort to being called a doctor. A great many of them make this decision on the rebound of being unaccepted by medicine. As you know, deciding on rejection is not always wise.

Possibly over one half of students who enroll in chiropractic schools each year are rejected medical school applicants. They wanted to be doctors and still want to be the doctor their mother and high school teachers wanted them to be. But the cold reality is, there aren't enough seats available. When I counsel students that have a high ambition of being a medic, I emphasize that they will be going up against at least 2,500 other students who are also seeking one of those 250 available freshmen seats. Then I ask them, Do you have a backup plan if they do not accept you? Not that I want their backup plan to be to switch to chiropractic school. I absolutely do not. If I were running the chiropractic school, I would encourage them not to become a chiropractor. Why? Think about it. Why would they want to be a second string? If you had your heart set on being a medic, would not chiropractic be demeaning? I would highly recommend these students go into a different science field. The brilliant students who were unable to get into medicine will likely be bored in chiropractic school. Chiropractic is one of those things in life that does not change. Our job is to keep the hips aligned, the sacral base level, and the spine straight. It is fantastic to see the impressive results we get from the repetitious work we perform. It is like going up to the plate and hitting a home run every time. However, you do the same thing over and over. I have observed over the years that this repetition drives the highly intelligent chiropractors up the wall. Science, technology, and medicine are always changing; the gifted students need that change factor to keep them interested. If they couldn't get into med school, they should be encouraged to go into engineering, research, or another aspect of science. These areas would dovetail with their intelligence and challenge of changing environments.

Chiropractic is a field for the B students that have to study a situation before making a decision. The B and C students tend to demonstrate more compassion and empathy as chiropractors for their patients. They usually tend to understand that life for many people is not easy. They possibly did not have it easy when they were studying complicated subjects. Most highly intelligent students never realize that B and C students, me included, had a darn tough time putting it all together. What I've witnessed over the years is, the B and C students will have more patience and perseverance than those that do not have to work at their studies.

Chiropractic is a field that requires a lot of good ole down-home common sense. Common sense is one of the laws of life that never change, but it has to be applied. Chiropractic is a field that requires physical work, and it has been my experience that physical work is below the pay scale for many with high intellect. It is not a field where you sit behind a desk and give out advice and wisdom. You have to physically adjust a person, which requires some shoving, pushing, and pulling. The highly intelligent chiropractors that I know are not really into this type of physical toil. Therefore, with these remarks in mind, I would highly recommend that valedictorians or medical "wannabees" of any class not go to chiropractic school. When Abner Flexner reorganized all the professional schools, he set up doctoral programs in all fields. Valedictorians and salutatorians may find challenging realms in areas more to their liking. School counselors should keep these statements in mind.

CHAPTER 21

Real Doctor versus a Chiropractor—What a Goal

Our problem today is the licensing laws that allow chiropractors to practice nearly any health discipline except for prescribing drugs, performing surgery, or dentistry. This open-door policy plays into the hands of the wannabe medics that wound up getting a chiropractic degree. Once they have their chiropractic degree, they work hard to make themselves look like a real doctor. To the chiropractors who entered the profession to be a chiropractor being a real doctor is not an issue.

Many times in the community, I have been asked, "When are you going to become a real doctor?" It doesn't bother me. I wanted to be a chiropractor. My educational background consists of a BS in education and a DC in chiropractic. This question bothers some of my colleagues who only wanted to become a chiropractor but do not have an undergraduate education. Many of the older chiropractors attended Chiropractic College straight out of high school. As time went by, the requirement of two years of undergraduate work was added, but they do not have a degree to fall back on, which makes them insecure. We will discuss later how not requiring chiropractic students to have a bachelor's degree has hurt the profession. In the meantime, the reality of not being a real doctor is an essential issue for the wannabees as they do not like being demeaned as not being a real doctor. They have fought for legislation to include sports medicine, physical therapy, acupuncture, oriental medicine, and a plethora of other therapies to give them the appearance of a real doctor. However, it is never enough. Now states like New Mexico and Wisconsin want prescription drug writing privileges. They want to pass out pills just like real doctors.

Currently, Wisconsin has written a bill that creates a new classification of health-care providers called the PSCP, or Primary Spine Care Practitioner. It is designed to address the growing burden of spine-related disorders and the overuse of prescription drugs. Its goal is to pursue the development of an expanded scope of practice for chiropractors. It will require five hundred additional hours of clinical study to allow the chiropractor to obtain a master's degree in PSCP. This degree will grant them the ability to order advanced imaging studies or procedures, along with the ability to proactively manage over-the-counter medications and pharmaceuticals.

Wait a minute, I thought the goal of this new degree was to address the overuse of prescription drugs. There appears to be a severe dichotomy here.

The "real" chiropractors are those of us who love to keep the hips, sacrum, and spine adjusted to restore and maintain the integrity of the nervous system while never claiming we treat disease. This is what a chiropractic adjustment does, and it works whether there is scientific evidence or not.

They Will Never Give Up

As in Wisconsin and New Mexico, the wannabe chiropractors want to be physicians with prescription rights. It isn't about helping people in the community. It is about their egos, their greed, and their envy of the medical profession and their place in it, which they could not attain.

Readers in Wisconsin and New Mexico should contact their state representatives and ask them to vote no on any prescription rights for chiropractors. There are many reasons they should not have these rights, but mainly when patients go to a chiropractor, it's because they want an adjustment, not a pill. However, before you vote, look in the 185th vol., no 22/2015, of Time Magazine. The front cover reads, "They're the most powerful painkillers ever invented. And they are creating the worst addiction crisis America has ever seen." It goes on, "Why America cannot kick its painkilling problem." The article states that an average of forty-six (now they say 150) Americans die every day from prescription opioid overdoses. They continue, "There are enough pills prescribed every year to keep every American adult medicated around the clock for one month." It's unbelievable that MDs are writing so many scripts that they could drug all of us around the clock for one month. I would say, follow the money as to why this crisis exists. It is an entirely man-made public health epidemic. The drug companies and the medics make big money pushing these drug medications. Why on earth would chiropractors want to add to this insanity other than for money? How can you be an honest doctor yet hand out pills like candy and live with yourself? The medics can get by with it because their stature in society is that they are godlike and can do no wrong. I would hope that my fellow chiropractors would not stoop so low as to want to help drug up our country any more than it already is. If you have a chance to look at the article, it is scary.

The profession, for the public's sake, has to deal with these wannabees who want to add drug use to the practice of chiropractic. They are outsiders who never wanted to be chiropractors, and they are pouring into the profession, much like the illegal immigrants flooding into the country. Instead of blending into and accepting our profession and culture, they want to keep theirs, and it is not working out very well for either.

Just like trying to develop two cultures in America that will never work, the chiropractic profession forming two cultures will not work. If it were, we would see 95 percent of the population rather than 5 percent. Chiropractic was designed to get you well and help you stay well. The wannabees try so hard to change the concept and mission of chiropractic that it messes up everything for the general public. They think only of themselves over helping you. They want to use medical therapies that possibly have nothing to do with your case to pad their bills. When you go to a chiropractor, you want an adjustment. They would rather push medical procedures on you versus adjusting you. Now they want to add drugs so they can help keep all of us doped around the clock. What a goal! I believe that should the chiropractic profession get prescription rights, half of the profession would never give another adjustment.

An osteopathic acquaintance of mine asked me, "When are you chiropractors going to get prescription rights? It is so much easier to write a script for the patient's pain than to get out of the chair and physically adjust them." He was brutally honest because adjusting a 250-pound patient is hard work. I am sure this is why the wannabees want to get away from adjusting because it is blue-collar work. Chiropractors that love to adjust do not mind hard work. However, for many cerebral people, hard work is not their cup of tea. Thus, there is a push to prescribe. So all of you in New México and Wisconsin, please vote no when this issue comes up in your state. Heaven knows we have too much addiction already.

Get your kids hooked on adjustments rather than drugs! Teach them to be like Uncle Gene. When he got "out of fix" with one hip high, he went to the chiropractor instead of taking medicine.

CHECK THE KIDS

Cars and kids, neither work right when they are out of alignment.

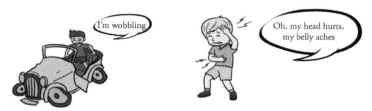

Cars and kids go like 60 when they are in alignment.

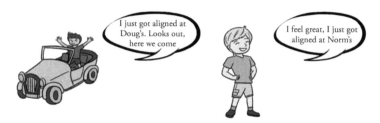

Check your kids alignment regularly. When hips are out of alignment, take them to the chiropractor. Straight spines and level hips make for a healthy kid.

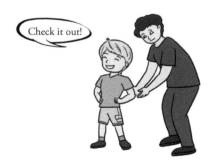

The Third Reformation—
Vendors and Practice Builders

CHAPTER 22

Jimmy Parker

The next reform that should take place in the profession deals with vendors and practice builders. Since we currently cannot write prescriptions or have the 1:1,200 ratio of guaranteed patients and other perks the medics have, it is difficult for many chiropractors to make it in practice. It is challenging primarily from acrimonious policies the chiropractic profession promotes. The profession has directed the chiropractors to use all sorts of therapies on patients rather than adjusting them. Most patients seek chiropractic care for an adjustment, not wanting, much less desiring to pay for other therapies. Patients want an effective adjustment at an affordable fee. Instead, the chiropractor is being trained to force therapies on you and charge exorbitant fees. With high prices, the chiropractor has to become a great salesman to survive. Some authorities say only 50 percent of all chiropractors make it after five years of practice. This predicament opens the door for practice builders. What are practice builders? They turn a humanitarian chiropractor who went to school to be a loving, compassionate caregiver into a high-powered salesman. Unfortunately, in chiropractic today, most chiropractors have to take courses from practice building groups and become high-pressure salesmen to survive.

Enter Dr. Jim Parker

Practice building in chiropractic along with the other five reforms that need to take place are directly related to the reason the profession sees only 5 percent of the population. This movement started in the late 1940s by Dr. Jim Parker from Fort Worth, Texas. During this period, chiropractic was trying desperately to get back on its feet. The profession was still reeling from the devastating beating the medics and the government administered to it during the twenties. They tried to jail chiropractors and forced them out of business for practicing medicine without a license. Thankfully, the public demanded the legislatures give chiropractors licenses. The people knew it worked, and whether it was scientific or not didn't matter. By the 1940s, close to 80 percent of the states had some licensure in place to allow chiropractors to exist, but it was a slow process. Incredibly, it would take another twenty years before all the states offered protection.

The 1920s to the 1940s was a horrible time for chiropractors. It could be compared to the Jewish people in Germany when the Nazis came looking for them. Chiropractors had to live underground and keep on the move. They could not put out their shingle. They ran their practices out of backrooms, much like a speakeasy during prohibition. A password or name of the person that referred you was needed to enter.

I was in high school from 1954 to 1958, and the chiropractor my family utilized had to move four different times. We followed him until the early1960s when the medical examiner finally caught up with him. Since he did not have a license, they made him stop practicing. It was sad because he was a great adjustor helping people who came from all over for his service. The worst part is that Indiana got its license in the midsixties. If only he could've hidden out for a few more years.

Once chiropractic licenses were in place to protect the chiropractor and the public, they were able to begin rebuilding the profession. Dr. Jim thought it needed to be accomplished faster and he was going to find a way to "pull the chiropractors up by their bootstraps."

Chiropractic flourished from 1904 until the middle 1920s, with more than thirty thousand chiropractors spread across the country. Chiropractic was founded in Davenport, Iowa, in 1895 by DD Palmer. In 1904, BJ Palmer, DD's son, started the first successful chiropractic school. In six months, utilizing an eight-hour study day five days a week, you could become a chiropractor. The Palmer's uncovered a simple concept and a vitally important fact; to keep anything in operation (e.g., a door, a window, a car, or any machine) they all have to have proper alignment. They taught that the atlas—which is at the base of the head, the vertebrae, sacrum, and pelvis—all need to be in alignment for proper nerve/blood flow for mobility and good health. This part of the curriculum was simple, and it is just common sense that spinal alignment is necessary. The complicated part was learning how to adjust the vertebrae properly. Acquiring the skills of adjusting is the key to being an excellent chiropractor. The Palmer's school concentrated on this by making the students practice over and over. By focusing more on skills and becoming very proficient at adjusting, fantastic results occurred. Chiropractic spread like wildfire from 1904 to the 1920s. Then the massacre by the medics and government took place. However, the medics and government could not drive us out of business entirely, but they still found ways to have an input on licensing. They made us study masses of medical material that have no relation to chiropractic. The time needed to teach the repetitive skills as were done at the Palmer school was set aside. One reason chiropractors use all manner of therapies today is that they cannot get results with only their adjusting.

The result of these dramatic adjustments early chiropractors produced got patients so excited they sent in their friends and family. This excitement would spur someone whose condition was resolved by the chiropractor to say, "Hey, how do I become a chiropractor? I want to help people like you helped me." The chiropractor would send them to Davenport, Iowa, to the fountainhead.

Thirty thousand chiropractors were produced in sixteen years, which is pretty amazing since there was no high-speed internet. It was unbelievable results along with positive talk about what the chiropractors were accomplishing that made it happen. Among the enthusiasm and great conversation, eavesdroppers heard all this excitement. It ruffled the feathers of the medics who saw themselves as gatekeepers, and it was not long before sides were chosen and the war began.

The medics realized that something had to be done about these upstarts. The success of these quacks could not be allowed. Health care was the medics' bailiwick, and they were not going to let anyone give them competition.

They mounted, and I mean *mounted*, a campaign to wipe out chiropractors. Their modus operandi was to arrest all chiropractors for "practicing medicine without a license." The result was nearly obliterating practicing chiropractors because chiropractors had no laws to protect them.

When the medical/government and Carnegie Institute reorganized education and developed the laws that created the proclamation that there would be only one medic per 1,200 in the population, those issues stabbed the heart of the chiropractic profession. This entire plan: education, laws, and the 1:1,200 ratio was said to be put in place to "protect the public." This false narrative was precisely to protect medicine from anyone that would give them opposition and competition. During the first two hundred years, our country had freedom, but these freedoms began to contract with the inception of this closed-door policy. During this time, the medical profession became the most powerful union in the country and still is to this day.

Upon implementation of their plan, the medical directors for the state began rounding up chiropractors. They used the sheriff and their deputies to invade every city and town where there was a known chiropractor. The chiropractors were ordered to cease and desist. If they did not, they were arrested and went to jail.

By 1930, the thirty thousand chiropractors that were practicing in 1920 had dwindled to five thousand. Wow! Their scythe mowed down three quarters of the chiropractic population. It took a lot of spirit to stand up to these bullies, but chiropractors felt compelled to help patients. Fortunately, enough chiropractors evaded, hid, or moved around fast enough to stay ahead of the posse and showed the medics they were not going to destroy their profession. Chiropractors knew adjustments worked, and it would be wrong to let the ailing public suffer solely for the greed of the big guys, not wanting competition.

It was entirely due to the grit and courage of a bunch of stouthearted chiropractors that chiropractic survived. In time laws started being passed in several states, and by the 1940s, the profession was turning around. It was at this time that Dr. Jim Parker stepped in to help out the profession.

CHAPTER 23

Salesman Extraordinaire

The Palmers were correct in introducing structural integrity as vitally important to good health. In the thirties, the first laws for chiropractors were enacted that would help protect them from the state's medical boards. It was during this "hanging on by the fingertips" atmosphere that Dr. Jim Parker developed his famous practice building procedure that still exists today. He believed that if chiropractors could make more money that would help them become more acceptable to society. They needed stand-alone offices to get out of backrooms and speakeasy environments to change the image of the profession. By all means, it was essential for the chiropractor to drive a Cadillac; he also thought they needed to join country clubs to project their image of success. The question was how to make the chiropractor into a financial icon in the community.

Dr. Jim had the solution, which he laid out in two parts; first was the three-day examination, and the second was the written report. Assume that you are a new patient entering Dr. Jim's office. You would first fill out a standard personal health form. Next, you would go to an examination room for a case history and physical exam. After the history and exam, you would be informed that X-rays are necessary. (The next step is vitally important to make Dr. Jim's procedure work. It is a line that Dr. Jim emphatically stressed must be stated.) "Because there definitely may be something wrong with your spine that could be causing most, if not all, of your trouble, we need to determine if you are a chiropractic case."

After the X-rays are taken, you will be told there will be no treatment today. The doctor will need time to analyze the films and results of your exam. You will be given a urine bottle to fill overnight and return to the front desk.

At the front desk, an appointment will be scheduled for the following day. You will then be asked to pay your bill. For hypothetical and simple figuring, let us say Dr. Jim is charging $250 for X-rays and fifty dollars per visit. The receptionist will have been coached to say, "That will be $300 today, would you like to pay by cash or check?" In those days, they needed to collect this first fee. This fee is called the EAR fee. EAR is an acronym for entrance, acceptance, and retainer. The *retainer* is the critical word here. Besides the urine bottle to collect your sample, you are also given another health questionnaire to complete and bring with you the next day.

On the second day, you arrive at the office with your urine bottle and filled out health forms. You are escorted to an exam room and asked to put on an exam gown because more tests and X-rays are needed. The testing today includes neurological, orthopedic, and kinesiological tests, which will be given to correlate with yesterday's and today's X-rays.

After these examinations, you will again be told, "There will be no care given today because it is still too early to determine whether you are a chiropractic case."

Remember, I previously stated that anyone is a candidate for chiropractic care as long as they have a spine and structural deviation. To make Dr. Jim's three-day examination and written report work, Dr. Jim saw that he had to place a moderate to severe amount of gravity on this issue.

Once the second day's exams are over, you return to the front desk, where the good news is that there is no charge for today's visit. Here you are informed that your next appointment is very, very important. The doctor will explain the findings of your case, and you must bring your spouse along for the report of findings.

On the third day, you and your spouse arrive at Dr. Jim's office. You are escorted into a beautiful plush office. The assistant will seat you in comfortable chairs and hand you the famous blue book with its report of findings.

First, the booklet will state that you are a chiropractic case. Of course, the chiropractor knew this from the beginning because you have a spine. However, to make this milking-room procedure work, there is more. The second part of the report explains how chiropractic works. Thirdly, there are blanks in the blue book report that have been filled in by Dr. Jim as to how much time it will take for you to recover and, the best part, how much it will cost.

The summary of findings may look like this:

A. Because of the severity of the case, it will take approximately 15 weeks to solve your problem.

B. You will need to be seen three times a week for the first five weeks.

Followed by two times per week for the next five weeks and finally once per week for five weeks.

C. The charge is $50 per visit, a total of $1500 for your case if you pay for each visit at the time of service. However, if you pay for all of your visits in advance, we will discount it 30%, and the amount you pay today is $1050.

Dr. Jim would give you plenty of time to read and digest the part in the booklet that states, "Yes, we can help you; you are a chiropractic case." Ordinarily, the patient will soften to the dollar amount and amount of time it will take to solve the problem by the time Dr. Jim entered the room. Hopefully, the patient is ready to sign on the dotted line and begin care.

Dr. Jim was adamant about issuing this report because he said it was the way medical doctors play the game. He saw the medics send patients for several tests. When the results arrive, they approach the patient and say, "Mrs. Jones, the tests show that your gallbladder has to be removed." It is not the doctor saying that the gallbladder has to come out—the test says so. Who can argue with tests? It takes the responsibility off the doctor's back. Thus, Dr. Jim's blue book, or his report of findings, is based on the two-day examination and tests. Tests show that you need thirty visits in fifteen weeks to solve this problem. It is not Dr. Jim saying this, but the tests!

In Dr. Jim's classes, he will teach the chiropractor all the right words and phrases to use to get the patient to buy the extended-care package. Knowing how to sell the patient on extended care was thoroughly taught by Dr. Jim in his Parker School of Professional Success. To be financially successful, the chiropractor needs to convince the patient to write a check for the 30 percent discounted amount of $1,050 today. Getting the check will assure the chiropractor that you will follow through with your care. If you discontinue care after three or four visits, it makes a nice profit. A refund is generally not requested or offered.

The profession started getting back on its feet and becoming financially successful in the sixties, primarily due to Dr. Parker's procedure. The better the chiropractor was at setting up the three-day routine and the more polished they became at selling the report of findings, the more dough they put in their pockets. The Parker Procedure was putting many chiropractors in the $100,000 a year income bracket in the late sixties, which is nearly three quarters of a million dollars today. The Parker School of Professional Success became the most popular entity in the profession. Believe it or not, it still maintains its swagger today, some fifty years later. There are nearly sixty practice building companies in the country today, and the Parker School remains one of the most popular. Parker is based out of Dallas, Texas, and holds a four-day session four times per year. It does change its venue to different cities on occasion, but it always keeps its January seminar in Las Vegas, where it may draw four or five thousand chiropractors. Instead of the $100,000 practices, today they talk of 1-million- or 2-million-dollar practices. No wonder they are popular if they can teach you how to make that kind of money.

You are probably getting the picture of why practice building is rampant in the profession. Chiropractic is not like the medical profession that has the billion-dollar pharmaceutical industry pushing drugs to patients. Drug ads are convincing you that you are sick. Medical doctors do not have to work hard to make a living because of the closed shop system. The medic is guaranteed 1,200 patients right out of school and has a billion-dollar drug advertising program running ads for them. The medical doctors can have the worst bedside manner in the world and still get by with it. They do not need to get anyone well; they can string patients along forever and have a financially successful practice. Plus insurance reimbursement was built for them, and they are practically guaranteed payment with no questions asked. Chiropractors have none of the luxuries the medics have. If the patient does not get well in the chiropractor's office, the patient does not come back and will not refer others. Medical doctors do not have to sell their patients on what they do. Chiropractors have to sell patients on care and what chiropractic can do. It is a burden, especially if you went into chiropractic for the sole purpose of helping people. Thus, having to sell is a thorn in the chiropractor's side, especially for the humanitarian-positioned chiropractor.

A dynamic adjustment can have the patient in and out of the office in just a few visits. Unfortunately, if they do not get results right away, they are out the door in the same one or two trips. If the chiropractor is charging a high fee for the adjustment, it is especially true.

Let us compare two patients with identical lower back conditions. One goes to an orthopedic surgeon who operates on a bulged disc. He trims off a piece of the disc that is bulging. Let us say the cost of this procedure is $20,000. The second patient comes into my office with the same condition. We align the hips, level the sacrum, and reduce the subluxated vertebra that is pushing on the lumbar disc. This procedure would take four to seven visits over two or three weeks and cost $120 to $150. In 80 percent of disc cases seen in chiropractic offices, the time frame is similar. The cost may vary, but it will never reach $20,000.

There is a constant discussion in the chiropractic profession as to why should not the chiropractor be paid an equivalent amount. If the results are the same, why is there such a discrepancy?

Additionally, the medics do not align the hips, level the sacrum, or correct the subluxated vertebra, all of which are instrumental in pushing the disc out in the first place. If these are not corrected, trimming of the disc will usually last only a few years—what a shocking fact for the excessive amount charged for trimming a disc. If you have had a disc trimmed and are experiencing symptoms, it's okay to go to the chiropractor to get checked. Chiropractors need to align your hips, level the sacrum, and check for subluxations of the fifth lumbar vertebrae so you will not have further rupturing. Your misalignment was possibly the reason for the rupturing in the first place, and a surgeon who trims the disc will never address what caused the problem. Chiropractors allow the body to return to normal without any visible evidence. There is no hospital stay and no scars. Without that visible evidence, the value of the chiropractor's work is unappreciated. However, having your body permanently altered by acquiring a significant, often grotesque, scar that you can show off at social gatherings, now that is worth big money!

Herein lies the frustration of chiropractors. Again and again, they pull patients out of some terrible health problems only to be paid a pittance in comparison to the medics. It is frustrating! The medics are white-collar thieves because they have no competition and can get by with it, period.

Dr. Jim Parker was upset about this when he set out to peddle his practice building idea, and it caught on like wildfire. It worked, especially for patients with chronic conditions who did not respond to medical care. They bought into Dr. Jim's report of findings, which offered hope, and usually, the cases the chiropractors accepted did get results. Patients would pay the upfront payment for those two to six months of care, and if the chiropractor could get two or three contracts per week, wow, that was money in the bank! Chiropractors were able to buy Cadillacs, join country clubs, raise their self-esteem, and produce a lot of wealthy chiropractors. However, in terms of helping most of the population, it left us seeing only about 5 percent, which is what we still see today.

Dr. Parker found a great way to assist the chiropractor gain wealth. Nevertheless, for every good deal, each party in the transaction has to come away, feeling they received something beneficial. Dr. Parker's idea should have had two equal parts, one for the chiropractor and one for the patient. Unfortunately, with his system, the patients always came up on the short end of the stick financially but not that they did not receive help because chiropractic is effective 80 percent of the time. Here is the reason; when Dr. Parker sold a thirty-visit plan, the patient paid the money for the whole course of thirty visits. What happens when the patient is better after three visits? The long-term plans are great to bring money into the doc's bank account, but handling the time frame is a nightmare. The only way this can work well is for each patient to get a little better on every visit. At the end of the contract, each patient is 100 percent recovered. Rarely is this going to happen because each person and each case is different. Dr. Parker's procedure puts everyone in the same treatment plan.

It would be prudent to assume that 80 percent of the people who buy a long-term Parker plan will get results, and most will get good results. If it is true when I state 80 percent of the people do receive suitable adjustments and respond very positively, why is it that only 5 percent of the population goes to chiropractors? This situation has been an enigma for the profession. Well, here are one or two of the reasons. When a patient goes to a practice building chiropractor, 80 percent of the time it will be a bittersweet experience. Most of these chiropractors make the cardinal sin that renders them impotent in their ability to attract new patients. They never release a patient. I'm sure you have all heard the biggest gripe about chiropractors, "The chiropractors make you come back forever!" It is the biggest slam about the profession. Chiropractors retain the patient far too long after the patient has responded and healed. The patient needs to be released when they feel good and are excited about what has happened. The chiropractic profession incessantly cannot let their patients go. They keep them coming back to milk as much as possible out of each patient. It is a malignant addiction the profession is saddled with and cannot throw off. If patients are not released shortly following feeling great, their enthusiasm rapidly dwindles almost to the point of bitterness if they are forced to continue. Even though they get great results, there becomes a haze over those results. Patients feel pushed into something they no longer think they need. You all have been in a situation where there becomes too much of a good thing. If forced to return, you are not going to be excited about referring any of your friends or relatives to the chiropractor. The chiropractor does a great job, and the patient likes the chiropractor personally, but the patient will never send them any referrals.

Most people who get good results but are hounded to come back again and again will not say much to anyone. Even though they feel much better, they will not encourage friends, relatives, or coworkers who may have a similar affliction to try their chiropractor. They do not want their friends to get into the same trap they got into, so they stay silent.

CHAPTER 24

They Will Never Let You Go

You never see chiropractic talked about in the media in any form. You do not hear people talking about it on the street. It is just never discussed; it is genuinely a faceless profession. Despite this, there is still enough influence to take care of twenty or thirty million patients per year, even with all its faults.

Chiropractic, as a profession, is a paradox. It is incredible that we can see so many people and yet never be discussed or talked about in any venue. A patient's great results never get any headlines, and generally few referrals are made. So how does it survive?

Chiropractic survives because it works! Unfortunately, the chiropractors and their management of the patients is what screw it up. When there are no referrals from their successes, chiropractors have to work at getting patients in their office. Most of them have to resort to advertising and soliciting for new patients. Advertising brings in another new patient, they get good results, and the cycle starts all over. The chiropractor cannot let go. They have to keep the patient coming back; it is like an addiction. The patient is excited, they are feeling much better, but the chiropractor cannot let go of this patient. They say to themselves, "When I felt that miracle happen, I was ready to go and tell the whole world. It was fantastic, but by being pressured to return after I felt so good caused me to sour on this great experience." Now, when anyone talks about health problems to these patients, they know where they could go, but instead, they are noncommittal. It is a story we all have heard, and it is disappointing it has turned out this way.

CHAPTER 25

Borrowing Money

Have you ever loaned money to someone and they had a tough time paying it back? It creates hard feelings, correct? Most authorities will tell, you are never to cosign a note for someone because most of the time, you will be stuck paying it. Well, the chiropractors have been borrowing money from their patients using the Parker procedure for years. Most business persons will say, you must put a product customers are satisfied with in their hand at a price they are willing to pay. You, the business person, are agreeable to let go of the product at a price that will satisfy you. Therefore, both parties are happy, both gain equally, and both are pleased with this exchange. Under these circumstances, people get excited about doing business with you. But in today's chiropractic business world, the chiropractors want the money upfront before they ever deliver you the goods or a product. The chiropractor's way of doing business is to ask you to pay them $1,500 upfront, which essentially is borrowing your money through their treatment program. Once they get that in their pocket, they will then start to deliver the goods. They do not provide it all at one time but rather every other day by you visiting their office over the next three to six months. The big difference between the chiropractor and the shopkeeper is that the shopkeeper sells you a tangible object, while the chiropractor sells you a "promise" with no guarantee that the promise will come true.

After the chiropractor accepts the "loan" of $1,500, there is an 80 percent chance of chiropractic helping you. There is also a 20 percent chance that you will not see the improvement you hoped for. Therefore, in all likelihood, there is a 20 percent chance of you getting stiffed on your loan to the chiropractor. The 20 percent who get stuck by putting out $1,500 without getting any improvement, along with the patients who got help but were coerced into coming back, add up to some pretty unfavorable numbers. It is not chiropractic that is at fault for the profession only seeing 5 percent of the population. It is their faulty patient-management schemes. They do something great, then turn around, and shoot themselves in the foot time and again. Eventually, you would think their foot would get sore.

Practice building companies have helped chiropractors by putting more dollars in their pockets. Dr. Parker's goal of the 1940s of pulling chiropractors up financially by their bootstraps has succeeded, but it has done nothing for you. The majority of you cannot get into a chiropractor's office because of the high costs. Potential new patients have no idea what chiropractic does because no one is telling them that structural health is just as important as chemical health. Today only chemicals are applied to our health problems. Most of these chemicals lead to more health issues. Also, the cost of chemical care is prohibitive. Presently the government is trying to step in and tell us that they will take care of all health care problems and costs. You know how that will turn out. The government will not add structural health care because they are in "cahoots" with the drug companies. As long as structural care is excluded from national health-care plans being proposed, the public will be left out again. A considerable portion of your paycheck will go for taxes to pay for everyone else's chemical care and drug addictions.

Chiropractors are the answer to the health care crisis that exists in this country. If chiropractors saw 80 percent of the population of the US, health care costs would ratchet down so fast that it would be unbelievable. Why couldn't this happen? In a word, *competition*. Competition drives the price of anything down. Yes! Competition and chiropractors could do it. They are the only ones who could give the medics competition since the osteopaths are now in bed with the medics. There are only three primary health care professions—medics, osteopaths, and chiropractors. But the big kicker is the 1:1,200 ratio that we have already mentioned. If the medics cared to lower health care costs, they could reduce the ratio and put more doctors on the street. Fat chance that will ever happen, so it is up to you, you and the chiropractors. Do you hear that, chiropractors? The public wants an adjustment, period.

If adjustments are not available to make you feel better, this exercise might be of some help.

DOG BALL

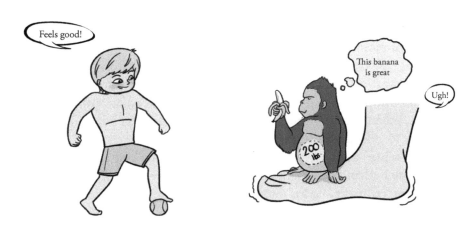

Rub your feet on one before you go to bed.

It breaks up the compression and fixation you create from standing all day.

If you were your feet, would you like a 200 pound gorilla setting on you all day?

Your feet are the farthest body part from the heart. This trick helps to irrigate the feet before bed.

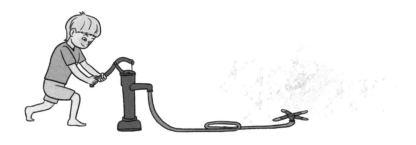

National Debt and Patriotism

Are chiropractors interested in you and your health? Are the chiropractors concerned and patriotic enough to help lower health care costs? Are chiropractors interested in lowering the national debt by helping to reduce the high cost of health care, which is one of the most significant reasons the debt is so high? They should be! Chiropractors have the knowledge and talent to reduce the health care costs in this country drastically. If enough chiropractors are aligning hips, leveling sacrum's, and keeping spines straight at affordable fees, patients will be glad to exchange a fair amount for chiropractic service. They will beat a pathway to chiropractic's door.

Presently the answer is no. The profession is not interested in helping all humanity. Their interest is in collecting eggs from the golden goose (government and insurance industry) or borrowing money from patients on the Parker plan. When a student enrolls in chiropractic school, they have a high ambition of learning to adjust and help a million people. Instead, the school washes those ambitions and ideas out of their heads and replaces the humanitarian chiropractic philosophy with medical indoctrination. The hopeful chiropractic student is educated into a quasimedical doctor so they will be acceptable with third-party payers. Their hope is for the chiropractor to be acceptable in all social circles. They're not interested in helping others. It's similar to Congress when they promise to help all of us, but once they get to Washington, they forget their promise. So be it with the hierarchy of the chiropractic profession—they care less about helping patients or being patriotic and trying to help lower healthcare costs.

Chiropractic, on the other hand, teaches students that they should be able to enter the field, build a two-million-dollar practice, and go to the top immediately. Chiropractors see the medics grow a great practice instantly. But our profession forgets that the medics have 1,200 people waiting in the wings along with the drug companies giving millions of dollars in free advertisements. The chiropractic students are thrust out in the world without 1,200 patients waiting or with free advertising. There is an estimate that 50 percent of all chiropractic graduates leave the practice of chiropractic after five years, and this is a crying shame. The hierarchy of the chiropractic profession should be "drawn and quartered," as the old saying goes. Our educational system is allowing half of our graduates to walk away at the end of five years, and the rest are only seeing 5 percent of the population.

Practice Builders Step In

Because chiropractic schools are failing to prepare the chiropractor for what the public wants from a chiropractor, an excellent adjustment, we also have this dreadful 50 percent dropout rate in the profession. This becomes fertile ground for the practice builders to step in and teach the remaining chiropractors how to make $2 million each year. The practice builders primarily show the chiropractor how to sell the patient on chiropractic services because they are sales gurus. If chiropractors master the ability to sell, they will succeed in chiropractic today. The student that has a humanitarian desire to help people but is not cut out for the sales force becomes one of the 50 percent who drops out. The sad part is that they are usually the ones who have compassion and empathy for people who are down and out and need help. Unfortunately, the chiropractors that are dropping out are often the ones who would make the best adjustors and healers.

If chiropractors learn the sales know-how, the practice builders will show them how to make it big financially, by preying off the backs of a few chronic patients that have outstanding insurance or the financial ability to "loan" the chiropractor money upfront for their care. Most of the chiropractors in the country use one or more of the sixty practice building companies. The majority of the companies use some of Dr. Jim Parker's format. Most of the patients who are cared for by chiropractors in this country are the chronic ones who have been everywhere with no results, and chiropractic is the last resort. This patient is a gleam in the salesperson's eye because they can be sold a bright-red porch swing even if they don't have a porch.

CHAPTER 26

Turf Wars

My practice is different. I charge a fee any patient can afford, and I accept patients without an appointment. When my patients ask for a referral because they are moving or they know someone in another state who needs an adjustment, I have no answer. I know that most of the chiropractors will want to set them up for a case plan that expects upfront money. In reality, most of the patients will continue to not have access to a chiropractor giving affordable adjustments for significant improvements in health, which we all need from time to time. I am sorry, but I do have good news that I will share with you in more detail later. There is a sensible educational plan that can be implemented to help the public. This approach would not eliminate the practice builders and procedures used by them or chiropractic/medicine physicians. It would reduce the stranglehold on how chiropractic care is practiced and controlled.

The medical profession has only one head organization telling them how to run their profession. In the chiropractic profession, we have several entities that control how we practice. The turf battle is between these factions. There is the chiropractic educational system, the chiropractic/medical group that controls our schools, the national organizations, i.e., ICA, FSCO, ACA and numerous others, along with practice builders.

Chiropractic sees so little of the population but not because it does not work. Chiropractic does work; it works at an 80 percent satisfaction rate. Infighting and practice builder's sales programs are partially to blame. Five percent is a failure rate by all standards and has absolutely nothing to do with chiropractic's success rate. Constant fighting affects all of us because we, in the 95 percent group, have few places to go to get a gem of an adjustment.

The bickering between these various factions is another reason the profession is faltering in its obligation to the public. The practice builders do a great job of helping chronic patients get better results by keeping them under care longer. Mismanaging acute patients by trying to borrow money from them and not releasing them when they should, may taint many who could be referring patients to them. The chiropractic/medical wannabe group does not see as many patients as straight adjustment-only chiropractors. They have been taught to be akin to medical doctors but are licensed to enter the field to practice chiropractic. It can become a nightmare for many graduates, and it prevents them from succeeding in practice. This chiropractic medicine group lacks the understanding that (1) chiropractic is a simple concept and that they will never be able to change and make it a complicated medical entity and that (2) they need to get out and see what actual working people want, which is an adjustment so they can get back to work tomorrow. They do not want a "glenoid labial bursa tendonitis" type of diagnosis. Working people want an adjustment; they want it now, not tomorrow, and they want it to be affordable. Unfortunately, the chiropractic/medicine group will not relinquish their hold on the educational system because it gives them power at your expense.

The Fourth Reformation—The Insurance Industry

CHAPTER 27

Easy Street

How would you like to bring in two hundred dollars for ten minutes of gab? What a gig that would be. That is what most medical doctors do all day. Multiply that by six to eight patients per hour for six to eight hours. Chiropractors see medical doctors having this routine, and envy comes to the surface. Who wouldn't love to have a job like that? I am sure there is a little envy in all of us when we see people having more than we do. Since chiropractors are called doctors, why should they not have part of that gravy train? The chiropractic hierarchy is working hard to get chiropractic included in all government and third-party pay groups for this reason. The elites of the profession have the delusional mindset that they can attain the lofty heights of the medics. The wannabes in the profession are like the proponents of communism—it sounds like a great idea, but it doesn't work and never will.

The same is true with chiropractors. No matter how hard they try to get into the medical fraternity, it will never happen. But they will keep trying, and the public will be left hanging without having access to a beneficial, affordable adjustment. The hierarchy of the profession should check out the Ten Commandments; number 5 says to honor your father and mother, which implies that someone will always be above or better than you. Accept it. The tenth commandment states, you shall not covet—meaning, in this case, they have it, accept it, and if you want it, go to medical school and earn it as they did.

Comment

Chiropractors chose and committed to a profession that help patients. They have to use bodily exertion and physically adjust people. Chiropractors covet the hefty fee the medics charge and receive for a self-limiting condition. Sixty percent of medical patients would get over their condition if they stay home, take care of themselves, and use a little common sense. If you do not let a fever or sniffles run its course, you will never build up immunity against colds or flu. If you do not self-immunize, you will be running to the medic all the time. That is the nature of the game—keep people sniffling and keep them returning.

As the saga continues, the medics still get to sit at their desks and issue orders. For this patient, we will need an examination, blood tests, or other tests, and these can be done by the nurse or the lab down the street. Once the test results are in, the patient sits before the medic and will be issued a script to take to get the necessary pills for this particular sniffle. The patient returns home and dutifully takes their medicine.

What an excellent setup for the medic. They do not have to see the patient for two weeks or more. In most cases, they will not see them at all, because 60 percent of the cases are self-limiting. Pretty remarkable, eh? They receive a significant office fee, have no follow-up with the patient, the case is closed, and they go to the next sniffle.

Here is where the chiropractor has to accept the situation in where they find themselves in. It's a fact that the medic gives the medicine, and it or the treatment takes place out of their sight because the patient does it at home. The medic does not have to observe, listen, or partake in the process; they are still sitting behind their desk at the office or out playing golf.

The chiropractor, however, has to be physically involved with their patient's treatment. The patient has to come into the office several times to receive their adjustments. Giving adjustments is hard work. Today, possibly two thirds of all chiropractic patients are medical failures who have not responded to prolonged medication, surgery, or physical therapy. The chiropractor has to get up from his desk and physically adjust the patient to make their care effective, and most of these cases are not self-limiting. These cases have to be physically worked out. Chiropractors cannot be like the medics and push a piece of paper across the desk and tell the patient to go home. It is plausible as to why chiropractors get bent out of shape when insurance companies dole out big money to the medics for having put forth little effort.

Many of the chiropractors' cases are chronic medical failures, of which many will generally respond. But the patient has to come into the office for the physical adjustments, and the chiropractor will often have to put up with complaints about how they are not healing fast enough. A chiropractor hears this several times per week. In the medics' situation, if the patient is complaining about their care, they are at home and the doctor does not hear it. Besides, the insurance company will hassle the chiropractor for healing taking too long and not wanting to pay for the treatment. Maybe chiropractors have a right to complain about these issues. Compared to the chiropractor's job, the medics have it pretty easy. We have the same liability and responsibility as the medic but far more one-on-one investment in each patient.

CHAPTER 28

Oil and Water Do Not Mix

Unfortunately, there are many issues concerning chiropractic and insurance. First of all, chiropractic and acute catastrophic medical insurance do not fit because people do not go to chiropractors for broken bones. Catastrophic coverage originally was meant for the medics to care for trauma, fractures, and concussions. Eventually, insurance went from calamity insurance to standard treatment for any health issue. It was at this point chiropractors became upset and started working aggressively to be included in the insurance gravy train. It was a very tough fight for chiropractors to be accepted because insurance is the medics' ballgame, and they were not willing to share. With patience and perseverance, eventually, the profession found a way to get their foot at the door.

The world of insurance crept into the chiropractic profession in the 1970s, and it has been a nightmare ever since and is one of the reasons it needs to be addressed and corrected. This debacle of insurance coverage is another one of the reasons the profession only sees a trickle of patients.

Square Peg in a Round Hole

Chiropractic and insurance mix like oil and water. Insurance for all your health care (or should I say sick care?) is a terrible fit. Trying to fit chiropractic care into a medical mold is equivalent to trying to fit a square peg into a round hole. Insurance was initially established for catastrophic acts, problems beyond the family budget. Car insurance was instituted to cover severe issues that arise when you do not have money set aside to cover an accident. When you buy car insurance, they will pay for repairs that your car incurs during the coverage period. You must choose a deductible. Let us say you select a $250 deductible; you are then responsible for the first $250 when the car has a covered accident. With car insurance, you are responsible for changing your oil, aligning the front end, putting air in your tires, etc. But expensive accidents are covered minus the deductible. Health insurance was not designed to cover everything from the head, chest colds, runny nose, and ingrown toenails. Today it has morphed to the point where 60 percent of all doctor's visits are related to colds, flu, and respiratory problems. These conditions used to be taken care of at home with a dose of common sense. Unfortunately, most working mothers have no time to take care of their child at home, so off to the doctor they go for a prescription of whatever is popular today. These visits are what run up the cost of insurance. Medics are not going to complain; they love to have them come in because it's easy to push an expensive script across the desk. If they were honest, they would tell them to take two aspirins, drink plenty of fluids, and go to bed. Most of these visits are for self-limiting conditions that will go away in seven days with treatment and one week without it!

Back to the square peg in a round hole scenario. The insurance company argues for why they do not like to pay the chiropractor for multiple visits. It is because the medic examines their patient, makes a diagnosis supported by any number of tests, gives their recommendation, and sends them on their way. Chiropractors do very little of this. We have the patient return again and again; therefore, the insurance companies assume we are not as educated as the medics. The assumption is that we do not know what we are doing, which necessitates the patient returning again and again so we can figure it out. Therefore, the insurance company does not want to pay the chiropractor.

It was Dr. William Kelly, a chiropractor out of Plano, Texas, who figured out how to stop chiropractor's claims from being red flagged for nonpayment. He began teaching Insurance and Procedure seminars, showing chiropractors how to get the insurance company to pay them.

After studying and observing the insurance company procedures in paying medical doctors, he came to the following conclusions:

A) Medical doctor's services are 80 percent examination and 20 percent treatment.
B) Chiropractor's services are 20 percent examination and 80 percent treatment.

Dr. Kelly's seminars drew standing-room crowds of chiropractors in the 1980s because almost every chiropractor wanted to get in on the insurance bonanza. He would stand in front of his audiences and say, "Chiropractors, it is time, and it is a must to get away from treating people and get into the examination business." His criteria were based on the following: when Medicare came into being, the medics were told that if they proved that the gallbladder needed to be removed, they would pay for the removal. For example, when a medical doctor turns in a bill of $3,000 for a gallbladder operation, $2,000 of it is for the examination and diagnosis and $1,000 is for the removal. The case is closed, and the bill is paid. Dr. Kelly told the chiropractors that it is essential to bill higher for the examination than you do for treatment. Otherwise, it will look like you do not know what you are doing, and you will not be paid.

He explained that there are code numbers for each test. If you perform a test, you must list the code number and know how much each code is worth. Run enough tests to bring the examination bill higher than the treatment costs. If you do not get greedy, pad the bills excessively or try to fly under the radar of what they will pay, for each test code, you will have a good chance of getting paid. Dr. Kelly called this maneuvering slycology.

What Dr. Kelly accomplished when he urged chiropractors to assume the medical role and become diagnosticians was an opportunity for the chiropractors to get paid. They had to give up their principles for the silver of payment. There was a time when chiropractors did collect good money using slycology.

Along with Dr. Kelly's slycology, there is another procedure that the profession uses called slipstreaming. Many of you know what slipstreaming is especially if you are a truck driver. It is an area of reduced air pressure and forward suction behind a fast-moving vehicle. Truckers can save fuel by getting into the slipstream of another truck, while race car drivers save fuel for the final lap by slipstreaming the leader. The trucker or race car driver out in front is possibly not too happy with slip streamers. Slipstreaming works for those who may not be able to make it on their own, which is precisely what the chiropractors have done. Chiropractic and insurance are not compatible, but by Dr. Kelly flip-flopping the purpose of chiropractors and making them diagnosticians, the chiropractor is now paid by the insurance company.

The insurance industry was not ecstatic about adding chiropractic to their roles but was forced into it from laws passed by all state legislatures. Chiropractors were paid more with Dr. Kelly's slycology, but it was still not as much as the profession would like. Therefore, slipstreaming came about. Insurance would pay for a specified number of visits to the chiropractor. There was a limitation as to the amount of compensation on a patient. Since the profession has the broadest laws of all the professions, they can do almost anything under the sun except prescribe drugs, perform surgery, and pull teeth. Therefore, they discovered they could jump into other fields like physical therapy where numerous codes existed, which they could utilize and collect fees from. They even found they could slipstream the massage field. Remember, they do not want to pay chiropractors. But somewhere along the line, massage has been resurrected to a genuine medical necessity. It is now covered by most insurance. Chiropractors cannot get paid, but the old ladies of the night profession is now legitimate, scientific, and worthy of insurance coverage? The result is that almost every chiropractic office in the country now provides massage, and it will be paid for by insurance.

Dr. Kelly flip-flopped the chiropractor's agenda from primarily adjusting to performing examinations. The use of physical therapy as the primary mode of care and topping it off by giving the patient a massage is slipstreaming. They are utilizing someone else's effort for their gain. This is slycology, and it is pretty sly. Chiropractors have no remorse for slipstreaming the medics. Morally, living off someone else's gains would be shameful, but it doesn't faze the profession. I have never used insurance in my fifty-two years of practice because it can make you sly, devious, and dishonest. Chiropractors are not physical therapists. They are not massage therapists, and they are not diagnostic centers. The chiropractic profession has to sell its soul for pieces of silver to get paid handsomely. It bastardizes the profession with nonchiropractic therapies to get paid. Yet there appears to be no shame in doing so.

You may be saying, "Norm, you are hard on your fellow chiropractors." Maybe I am because they are freely using all these indirect methods to get paid handsomely. Other health care professions work the system for big money, too, and have no shame in milking taxpayers out of their hard-earned money. For example, a Medicare back surgery for $25,000 could be resolved with three or four visits to our office for one hundred dollars. Since Medicare came into being in the late seventies, no one has ever challenged the usage of all this testing until a recent article. In April 2015, there was an article written in the *Douglass Report* vol. 15, no.1, published by WC Douglass, MD, titled "The New Super-Bug Threat that You Need to Know About." He states that over five hundred thousand endoscopies are performed each year. He states these scopes are difficult to clean, resulting in bugs being transferred from one patient to another. Recently in Seattle, thirty-two people were sickened, and eleven eventually died from this contamination. In Los Angeles, some two hundred were sickened and two died. Other cities have also had outbreaks.

Dr. Douglass's primary point was the question, Are all these tests necessary? He states, and this is thirty-five years after Dr. Kelly told the chiropractors to get into the testing field; "The new gold rush in medicine isn't in drugs." It's in tests.

These days a lot of doctors will run every test in the book if they can get away with it. It adds up to some of the quickest cash in the business. They'll cram these tests right down your throat and up your you-know-what (and that is *not just* a figure of speech) whether you need it or not. Endoscopic tests use a camera on a tube to peek into your stomach, colon, intestine, and more.

Dr. Douglas continues that "while some of these tests can cost you (or your insurer) almost as much as a new car, the equipment they use can have more miles on it than an old Buick. Odds are that the old Buick might be a heck of a lot cleaner, too. Tubes that pass down throats and up countless rear ends to pick up the kinds of germs that hang out in those parts of town—and if you are unlucky enough to be on the business end of that scope during the next intrusion bugs from another patient could be passed along to you. It is a recipe for the superbug nightmare."

Dr. Douglass' s concern is twofold: (A) too many tests are unnecessary and utilized just to generate income, and (B) all those unnecessary tests result in a lot of unnecessary suffering. In my practice, I have had four healthy patients who went in for a routine scope. They wound up developing infections and passed away as a result of a perforated bowel, directly related to the colonoscopy. I am sure these four cases were not included in the numbers Dr. Douglass quoted.

Covering Our Backside

Mainstream medical doctors performing the majority of these tests will tell you that the problems the tests might create will pale relative to the issues they will find. They go on to say that it is essential to do all the tests so they will not miss anything. Have you ever heard a medic take the blame for causing a problem? It doesn't happen. They always have a reason to justify the situation. We have all heard how "the operation was a huge success, but the patient died!"

Because there is never any blame for a botched job, they, as Dr. Douglass points out, will run as many tests as they possibly can. Dr. Kelly was telling the chiropractors thirty-five years ago to get out of the treatment business and get into examinations because that is where the money exists.

However, chiropractors want to mimic the medics but are hamstrung because they do not have high-dollar testing machines. They have very few of the devices that rack up expensive examination fees that can cost the patient as much as a new car. The chiropractic profession is envious of the money the medics make on examinations and prescribing. Who can blame them? Look at the headlines of the October 6, 2015 *Wall Street Journal* vol. CCLXVI, no. 82. On the front page are these headlines: Price Increase Drive Drug Revenues. The article reads, "Demand for a drug called Avonex has declined every year for the last ten years." Well, this isn't "a problem for its manufacturer; the US revenue from the drug has more than doubled in that time, to $2 billion last year." Drug companies can boost prices even when the demand is not there. Of the thirty top-selling drugs sold by pharmacies, the revenue has outpaced demand by 61 percent. Unbelievable!

Wouldn't we all love to have our income increase 61 percent without working anymore or even working half as much? It is ridiculous how the medical world can raise prices on health care to generate enormous profits. The increase is only for the sake of profit and not for providing any additional service.

Envious as they may be, chiropractors have to accept the road they chose and make the best of it. Making big money is the medics' entitlement. They walled off their profession with the 1:1,200 ratio for the very purpose of not having competition. It is high time the chiropractic profession stops envying the medics and their insurance game. Chiropractic needs to do what it is designed to do—align the hips, level the sacrum, and straighten the spine. Give the patients an excellent affordable adjustment, and from personal experience, I guarantee that patients will beat a path to the chiropractor's door. The profession could flip flop from 5 percent to 95 percent. Well maybe not 95 percent, but it would undoubtedly be higher than the present 5 percent.

Millions and millions of people need help. What are we chiropractors doing? We are complaining that we are not getting entitlement and handouts like the medics. Chiropractic should not be spinning its wheels trying to become like the medics. It is a meat and potato's profession for working people. Chiropractic adjustments are needed by working men and women who make this country great. They should have the opportunity to have a chiropractor in their community who could give them an effective, affordable adjustment, getting them back to work in no time. They should not have to worry whether their insurance will pay for super high fees.

CHAPTER 29

Ideal Business Model—Not Being Used

Chiropractors have one of the best business models in the world. We have a product and procedure that can help everyone. Every person in the world needs chiropractic care at various times in their life, and it can be performed at a fair and reasonable price for everyone. Chiropractic is branded; most everyone knows that a chiropractor gives a spinal adjustment. Earlier I was saying the medics have it made with the 1:1,200 ratio, and they can come out of school and have a ready-made practice of 1,200 patients. Chiropractors don't realize the acres of diamonds they have. Medics only take care of sick people. Chiropractors take care of improperly aligned spines, hips, and sacrums for patients throughout their lifetime. What an opportunity for chiropractors and how beneficial for the entire world.

Instead of helping the world as they should be doing, chiropractors spend their time buying into schemes to learn how to make more money. Many of these schemes revolve around weight loss. In fact, many are advertised in chiropractic magazines such as *Dynamic Chiropractic*, which on June 11, 2015, included a four-page insert advertisement titled "Practice Success Today" vol. 12, no. 1, page 1. This insert was from the NuLean Company. It states, "A Gallup Poll in 2013 says that 51% of the public want to lose weight, and that weight loss presents a much larger market than chiropractic. By adding weight loss to your practice, you can increase your income from $10,000 to $150,000 per month."

Oh my goodness, $150,000 extra per month! When someone is selling that much per month, I doubt if there is much concern for helping you structurally. As I stated before, the successful chiropractors today are super salespeople. I used the analogy of selling the patient a porch swing even when they have no porch. How many patients coming to the chiropractor for an adjustment want to be converted into a weight loss patient? Typically, they are expected to buy an expensive $400 per month regimen of supplements that they have to mix in a blender. They will probably do it for two months and quit. Granted, people are overweight. Chiropractors will say it is their moral duty and responsibility to encourage the patient to lose weight for their health benefit. I get that, and so do most of you! However, where does the moral responsibility of being their chiropractor and selling patients $100,000 per month of weight loss powder run parallel?

Chiropractors have such a broad license. It allows them to do anything under the sun; it permits them to diversify and sell products not related to the chiropractor's brand. Chiropractors who are good salespeople can make fortunes selling health-related products. These same chiropractors will complain that they do not see enough new patients. Then they will spend huge money on advertising to attract more clients to sell more weight loss contracts. These chiropractors cannot get it through their heads that diversifying practices to include everything under the sun except adjusting is why we only see 5 percent of the population. How many patients went to a NuLean practitioner for an adjustment who happen to be a little weighty were sold ten cans of powder at eighty dollars per can by a good salesperson? The successful chiropractors today are very good at selling and are masters of the old bait-and-switch game. How many patients coerced into something that they did not want will refer anyone to that chiropractor? If you end up letting the chiropractor force you, you get upset with yourself. Even if the program works, you will not tell your friends or family about this chiropractor.

I take issue with these NuLean types of chiropractors who say that the weight loss program market is more significant than the chiropractic market. Hogwash. Everyone in the world needs chiropractic care throughout their life. As a practicing chiropractor for over fifty years and seeing a large volume of patients, rarely did someone come in not wanting an adjustment. If chiropractors would quit conning patients into all these other therapies and only charge a reasonable fee for the adjustment, we as a profession could be seeing over 70 percent of the population.

Unfortunately, chiropractic schools teach students that they need all these therapies to be successful. Did you notice I said "to be successful"? Then we have to determine whose success, the chiropractor or the patient?

Our educational system is not emphasizing that an adjustment is an intangible entity. They do not understand that when buying a product from a vendor, the product is something that you want or need and for which you are willing to pay a fair and affordable price. It is of benefit to both you and the vendor. Students coming out of school do not understand there is a ceiling on what the public is willing to pay for an intangible product that is not guaranteed. In my area, the average hourly wage for production workers is twenty-two to twenty-three dollars per hour. We have always set our fees at the area's average hourly production wage. It has been a good fit, the people love it, and we have been well blessed. However, when I see colleagues in the area double and triple that fee, there becomes resistance to paying forty-five dollars to sixty-five dollars. The chiropractor performs an intangible act, and the patient leaves the office with a hope and a prayer that it will work.

Chiropractic is an art and skill. To be a good chiropractor, you have to practice repeatedly to master both the adjusting art and the skill. I can understand why chiropractors say "we have greater skills than medical doctors." We do have an art and skill that no medical doctor will ever have unless they, too, spend countless hours developing the ability to adjust. We are doctors and have excellent qualifications. Ideally, we could say we should have the same status and pay scale as the medical doctor. Students coming out of Chiropractic College today believe that they are entitled and should be able to charge one hundred dollars per visit like the medics charge. But in real life, it does not work that way. The young graduate has no experience, their skills are questionable, and they are selling an intangible product with no guarantee. Our colleges are not being realistic with graduates when they send them out with this idea. It is evident that with no experience and dubious skills in addition to charging high fees, the patient will not come unless it is an absolute necessity. Usually, a six-pack or a bottle of aspirins will win out.

When a new chiropractor opens their practice charging one hundred per visit, other therapies come into play. This fee has to be "justified," and it is at this point, good salesmanship comes in. The patient enters the office for an adjustment, but the super salesperson converts that one adjustment into a series of twenty sessions of four or five different therapies and five cans of NuLean weight reduction powder. Maybe there will be an adjustment if they are lucky.

A little tidbit about America's favorite chair for backaches.

RECLINERS

Most everyone loves a recliner.

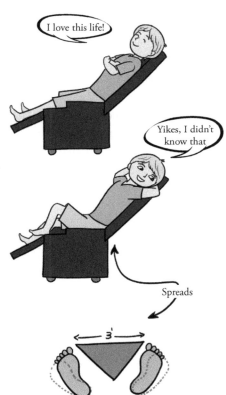

But, did you know your 'butt' widens with constant recliner use?

Recliner lovers will 'splay' their legs when leaning back to relax.

Constant flaring of the legs weakens the hip joints and "broadens your base."

My advice, burn your lazy boy and buy an upright wing back chair like your grandparents used.

Who Benefits?

When the colleges encourage graduates to leave school and go out to emulate the medics, who benefits? Well, for sure, it is not you. What you want is an adjustment, and most of you will not even attempt to go when the chiropractor has a one-hundred-dollar fee. If you do go and succumb to their sales pitch and go forth with their treatment plan, even if you get great results, you may wind up having buyer's remorse. Only 5 percent of the population is buying into chiropractors and their schemes. It is a crying shame that the profession has something so great to offer the world, which the public would utilize if it were affordable, but instead, they consistently play games trying to mimic and slipstream the medics to appear acceptable to insurance and third-party payers.

CHAPTER 30

Politics Government Insurance

There are politics in chiropractic as in any large organization. Socialism and entitlements have crept into chiropractic as well. In the voting populace of America, half want the government to take care of them, and the other half want to work and provide for themselves. Chiropractic is the same. Half want insurance and government programs to take care of their patient's bills. Insurance has deep pockets. If they can tap into those pockets, a lot of money can be made from their patient's care. The other half will adjust patients on a cash basis and work hard to make sure they provide excellent service so the patient will pay them.

In reality, insurance is nothing more than a redistribution of wealth. All of us pay into the insurance funds, but the fact is that 80 percent of the insurance money will be utilized by only 20 percent of the people. If we bake a big cake for one hundred people and only twenty people eat 80 percent of the cake, they would have tasted some large slices of cake, correct? Socialism at its best. Karl Marx, the author of *The Communist Manifesto*, which is the bible for communism and socialism, is very appealing on the surface. They tried to make it work in Russia. It did not fare well. In the end, the hierarchy got very wealthy, and the mass lived in two-room apartments. In America, the medical profession is set up like a socialist format, and who is getting rich? Who is using all the services? Who is paying these humongous bills for open-heart surgeries, hip replacements, etc.? You guessed it, you and I, the taxpayers. The medical profession is getting very wealthy off our backs. The chiropractors see this activity occurring and continue sidling up to the medics because they want to have a piece of that big cake.

The medics make massive salaries and receive fabulous fees from the insurance companies while they lie to the public and say they are overworked and underpaid. With government programs not allowing any more medics into the field and maintaining the 1:1,200 ratio, this restricts any direct competition for the medical and pharmaceutical companies. This way, they can charge anything they want, which is usually as much as the traffic will bear. By doing this, eventually, taxpayers will not have enough money to support their lifestyle. In Russia, this is what happened. The government cornered all funds, and finally, Russia went bankrupt.

Earlier, we discussed how chiropractors are borrowing money from their patients before they take care of them. The medics are doing the same thing. While the chiropractor is borrowing directly from the patient, the medics are borrowing the money from every taxpayer! At least when you loan money to the chiropractor, you are going to receive benefits from that money, but with the medics, only 20 percent of the taxpayers will benefit. We all send tax money into a fund hoping that someday if we have a medical condition, that money will be there to take care of us. Unfortunately, 80 percent of us will never use any of that money because 20 percent of the population uses 80 percent of insurance money.

For this reason, the medics can charge an enormous amount for their services. Remember the cake analogy I mentioned before? What a great situation for the medics. Taxpayers "loan" the government's and insurance companies' money through our taxes and insurance premiums. Then the medics get to dip into that big cake and take some pretty hefty pieces justified or not. People using tax and insurance money don't care how unreasonable the charge. They say, "Hey, insurance is paying. I don't have to pay. I don't care what gets charged. If the medic charges three times what it's worth, so be it."

It is so easy to use other people's money. The ratio that allows medics not to have competition protects them. As a result, they can accumulate great wealth. Most of us enjoy helping our neighbors, but few enjoy coercion to help them. Medics are no different than the socialistic communist party; they are reaping large rewards from the forced insurance premiums and government tax that burden all of us.

Interestingly, the medics have raised their fees so high that the cost of going to the doctor, even for a sore throat, is prohibitive without insurance. When a serious problem such as an operation arises, the price may be more than the worth of a person's house. Is there an ethical problem here? Even if there is, it appears no one cares as insurance caters to the medic's demands. If they want to be paid $100,000 for a procedure that could be done for six thousand dollars, there is no concern. If more medics were on the street, this would create competition, causing fees to drop. Unfortunately, the government, in its infinite wisdom, has decreed there is to be a health tax on everyone. All taxpayers can help pay the medic's outrageous $100,000 fee. Here you have socialism at its finest. National health care will not drop the cost of health care. All it does is guarantee that medics can continue to collect high fees from 20 percent of the population using the majority of insurance money. Is *bamboozled* the word for this course of action upon the public? They have coerced the taxpaying public by saying they will take care of all health problems. On the surface, this sounds great, but will we have any money left from our paycheck if patient after patient has to have a $100,000 operation?

The medics will not have to give up anything; they will continue to collect income that comes along with ill health. Government health care will be a mother lode for the medics. They will be able to accept all knee and hip replacements, heart and cancer cases, and conditions associated with sugar. They will not be limited to patients who can afford it through private pay or insurance. Isn't it interesting that 80 percent of these conditions are related to lifestyle and 80 percent of the insurance money will pay for these infirmities? Therefore, we taxpayers are being good Samaritans, and through our "lavish taxpaying contributions," we will contribute to helping care for our fellowmen. More than likely, they enjoyed overeating, smoking, drinking, and indulging in undisciplined activities resulting in enormous funds necessary to regain health.

The Old Testament says we need to render help when our neighbor's ox falls into the ditch. Nowhere in the Bible does it state we need to pull the ox out of his predicament while the owner sits on the sideline enjoying a seven-course meal. In my office, I ask patients who have had hip or knee replacements if the surgeon told them they should lose weight or change their lifestyle. Ninety-five percent say the doctor states they can go about their business as usual. Am I looking at this wrong, or are we taxpayers paying for the operation and contributing to seven-course meals that will foster more replacements?

Once It Starts

Once a government program starts, it will never stop. I imagine we will see more and more taken from our paycheck to pay for government health care. Just look around your communities. There are new hospitals, cancer centers, and health centers arising. It is known as the medical-industrial complex. Once it begins, it will never stop. In Great Britain, when Napoleon was on his rampage in Europe during the 1840s, the British government built outlook towers along the North Sea. Each was staffed around the clock so the army could be alerted if Napoleon was seen crossing the sea. Napoleon's threat came and went. He never did cross the sea, but the government towers remained. They were kept fully staffed for another one hundred years until they were destroyed when the Germans bombed England during World War II.

In the May 15, 2016, issue of *Dynamic Chiropractic*, possibly the most widely read magazine in chiropractic, the frontpage headline reads "Chiropractic Needs a Lesson in Education." The author, Dr. Steven Brown, states, "To achieve full physical status with Medicare, the chiropractic profession must increase its education and training requirements to compare with any other profession that has such status." The article is saying that if we increase our education and training, Medicare and private insurance could be mandated to cover all "medically necessary services" doctors of chiropractic are licensed to provide. Remember we mentioned earlier that chiropractic has a whole string of therapies that they perform in their offices, and this would be a giant step forward for the profession economically. It is all about money. Taking care of patients who need an adjustment is not mentioned. Sadly, helping others is not what is essential; it is the gravy train. The hierarchy knows as well as you and I that once a program begins, it will continue forever. Thus, we will have our Napoleonic towers.

CHAPTER 31

Forget Crumbs; Crumbs Are for Runts

Chiropractors do get some insurance payment from private and governmental agencies, but in comparison to the medics, it would be equivalent to crumbs off the banquet table. Time is spent filling out numerous forms and jumping through hoops to get those precious crumbs. They spend so much time filling out insurance forms they take their eye off adjusting patients and getting them back to work as soon as possible.

Presently, chiropractors are sitting on their talented hands, not using their abilities to help more of the public. They complain about not getting enough pay from their excellent work. They have been contributing to the government all along, and why should the government dole it out to a select few who use most of our health care money? We would all love to have some of our tax money that the government squanders each year returned to us. Let's be practical; once you give someone else your money, it is now *their* money. Hopefully, the chiropractors will wise up and realize they might as well quit sucking up to the medics hoping and praying for more than crumbs.

We are the runt of the healthcare world, eating leftover crumbs from the government and insurance programs. Someday, the profession has to accept the fact that chiropractors are separate and distinct. If the profession does not take a stand and change direction on our own, it will never happen.

The Vehicle

Chiropractic exists because of the adjustment; it is the vehicle that gives chiropractic the license to practice. Chiropractic is not a package of therapies. It exists to balance the hips, level the sacrum, and keep the vertebrae in the spine aligned. Therapies do not do this. Once chiropractors adjust their patients and provide them with considerable value, the patients will, in turn, provide the chiropractor with substantial wealth. It is as simple as that. Patients want an adjustment; they do not want all the nonsense chiropractors throw at them to run up a hefty insurance bill. Patients want a super adjustment at an affordable price. When that is delivered, everyone benefits. When this occurs, patients get excited, then they tell their friends, relatives, bosses, and coworkers. I guarantee that any chiropractor who serves their fellowmen in this manner will wish they had a clone. When the chiropractor uses the vehicle that makes chiropractic, chiropractic, both parties benefit, and it is suitable for all.

Lopsided Deal

Today, health care is lopsided in favor of medical providers. It is great for them; they typically get paid five hundred dollars or more per hour. But the patients do not necessarily get five hundred dollars' worth of care from the visit. The medic says, "Try this prescription, and if that doesn't work, come back next week, and we will try another." Even if none of the medicines work, the medics still get paid. They will receive $120 for your ten- or fifteen-minute visit. The medics get by with not practicing commerce like most other businesses. Typically, a company has to put a product in your hand that will benefit you and for which you will pay a fair price. The shopkeeper sets an amount that will satisfy his needs. Both parties are happy and benefit from the transaction. It is an equal give-and-take exchange.

Our current health care commerce system is very unbalanced. It stems back to medics having no competition and charging anything they want, whether it is suitable for you or not. How many times have you heard "If you do not have insurance, you will not get care for your condition"? When you go to a health care provider, what is the first thing they want to know—who is your insurance carrier? Shouldn't they first ask what your problem is? Unless it is an absolute emergency, they will want your insurance information. Wouldn't you love to have a job where there are hundreds of people waiting for you? You can make patients wait as long as you want because of no competition. You can charge anything you want because the money comes from an immense fund, deep as a hole to China. All of us would like that sort of a deal. Sorry, folks, it only exists in the medical field. They have a closed shop that very few can enter, and they have the insurance industry behind them. Unfortunately, we have, possibly foolishly, put our money in insurance. We lovingly help 20 percent of our neighbors who live a lifestyle conducive to problematic health, which, in turn, allows the medics to buy big cars and houses. Only a select few benefits in this lopsided health care scheme.

CHAPTER 32

Massage and the Real Doctor

Some years ago, to reverse the drop in applicants to chiropractic schools and to increase revenue, school administrators needed a plan. Like fast-food restaurants that add more items to their menu, some chiropractic colleges have added a massage school to their curriculum. Massage schools were incorporated into the curriculum, hoping to draw more people into the chiropractic environment.

The addition of more schools of study allows colleges to have university status. Now instead of being National College of Chiropractic, it became the National University of Health Sciences. We will discuss later how my profession isolates itself from the mainline educational system. It is trying very hard to become something more than spinal adjusters, but they will not ask for outside help to help them achieve this.

Hanky-Panky

With the sexual revolution that has taken place in the last thirty years, massage has become much more popular. It has, in essence, come out of the closet. It used to be that a massage parlor was where hanky-panky would occur. People would go in for a massage, and the fee for the massage would be posted. After the massage, you could ask the question, "How much for the other?" That fee was never displayed.

Today, massage has had a makeover. Its image has been cleaned up, and it is now called medical massage. It is chic to have a masseuse and spend fifty dollars a week on an enjoyable escape from reality. Massage is very relaxing and can soothe away much built-up tension that develops in our everyday lives.

Because of the newfound fascination for massage, a high percentage of chiropractors now offer massage therapy. It has become so legitimate that many insurance companies will pay for the service. It has become more legitimized than chiropractic. Listen to people on the street, in restaurants, workplaces, churches, almost anywhere, and you will hear them talk of massage, but not much about chiropractic.

Instead of having a sign in front of every chiropractor's office reading Adjustments Given Here, most have a sign saying Massage Therapy Available Here. It is rather humorous but sad at the same time to see the dichotomy. The profession is trying very hard to become scientific to be accepted and then to go all out for massage with less scientific credibility and its history of being associated with questionable issues.

Chiropractic brought massage therapy courses into the schools to increase student numbers and revenue. In the process, the schools and most chiropractors have found that the use of massage helps justify their high fees. Patients go to chiropractors to get an adjustment, but many are coerced into multiple therapies costing more than they wanted to pay. Therefore, to console you and make you forget about being conned into more than you wanted, the last thing you receive from a high-fee chiropractor's office is a massage to make you feel you are getting your money's worth.

CHAPTER 33

Twig in a Fence Row

When you go to the majority of chiropractic offices, there is no telling how many different services and therapies you will receive. Instead of concentrating on adjusting and getting children under care, they offer almost everything except an adjustment. In far too many offices, the adjustment is almost an afterthought. Think of a twig in a fence row. It will grow crooked if the fence is not pulled away, just as kid's spines become crooked from their various activities. How many young people grow into adulthood being out of alignment? Bones usually fuse around age eighteen. If the hips have not been aligned, the sacral base is not level, and the spine has been allowed to grow crooked, problems may develop. When they enter the workforce and begin heavy lifting and repetitive work, additional stress is placed on the body. The muscles will have enough tone for the first few years, but once the tone begins to diminish, joints will start to shift and problems will occur. Sadly, because we only see a small portion of the population, most people with hip misalignment and sacral base distortion will go to the medics. The standard therapy there is to take medication and a course of physical therapy.

Talk about twigs in a fence row. Look what the dental profession has done for straightening teeth. Beautiful teeth are great. I am sure straight teeth keep us healthier, give us more confidence, and make us feel better overall. But I have to ask, how much more important is a set of straight teeth than a straight spine?

There Is No Comparison

Just as a fence has to be straight and taut to do its job, so too with the spine. When a twig grows in a fence row, it alters the course of the twig and the course of the fence, and they cannot coexist and do their job correctly. The same situation occurs with children when one or two vertebrae subluxate in the spine, a hip misaligns, or the sacrum is not level. If a parent lets this go and does nothing to correct it before a child turns eighteen, those bones will end up malformed, which will create adulthood problems.

Many of you have spent a fortune on having your kids' teeth straightened, and they do have a great smile. Unfortunately, you did not have their spine straightened so they can have good health to go along with that great smile. Granted, you never thought about having their spine straightened, that is understandable, and I cannot fault you for that. My fellow chiropractors should be spending their time educating the masses that the spine is more important than teeth. They need to remove all the barriers that stop you from getting into a chiropractor's office. Orthodontists can charge an arm and a leg to straighten teeth and get away with it. Even though we can get by and live without teeth, it is usually an elected service.

Chiropractors are not in the orthodontist's fraternity. Because teeth are the first thing we see when we look at someone, we see those expensive well-aligned choppers. When chiropractors straighten a spine, it is hidden, and no one can see our work. It is tangible versus intangible. Yes, it is very frustrating to the chiropractor who saved a child from having a miserable life with three adjustments and gets paid one hundred dollars. An orthodontist receives $7,000–8,000, and it will barely affect the child's overall health other than having a great smile. How unfair is this? Chiropractors have to remember that they are a member of the chiropractic fraternity and that its job is to take care of intangibles. Intangibles will never have the value of tangibles.

Some Things in Life Have to Be Accepted

There is no comparison as to which is the most important; a straight spine is vitally more necessary than a pretty smile. Chiropractors are not seeing 95 percent of the population and not keeping spines straight. This becomes the main reason for many health problems existing today and why it costs so much for health care.

The chiropractic profession has to share a significant part of the brunt of the burden for this problem. My profession has one of the most exceptional vehicles to health, and one of the most significant responsibilities is to keep everyone in the world healthy. Chiropractic cannot be delivered to the public as other professions offer theirs. The medical and dental fields have a tangible item. They give medicine, leave scars, and straighten teeth. All are objects you can feel, touch, and observe, and people will pay for these tangible items. They have straight teeth and scars they can exhibit at the next social outing. These are delivered, substantial visible changes. Chiropractors provide the intangible. The patient may come in with a frown on their face from not feeling well and leave with a smile because the adjustment made them feel better. But they go out empty-handed. They go out with an intangible; they have nothing to show off at the next party. How can chiropractic patients compete with their friends showing off their scars and straight teeth? Chiropractors cannot compete with tangibles. We have to accept this!

CHAPTER 34

The Tipping Point

The tipping point has not been understood by the chiropractic profession. You can only charge so much for an *intangible*, especially if that intangible is not guaranteed. Our schools teach the chiropractic student that they are as good as any other profession, and I agree that what we do has tremendous benefits for the public. But they do not teach the intangible factor, which people will only pay out of pocket up to a point. There is a ceiling on what they will pay.

Patients will give you an excellent chance to help them if it is within their budget. If the chiropractor would conduct studies of the average incomes in their communities, they could get a feeling of what patients are willing to pay for intangible services. They do not want to pay for what your ego thinks you are worth. When a chiropractor understands where the community's fee ceiling is located and sets his fee at or below this amount, the public will beat a path to their door. They will come by the hundreds, but few chiropractors understand this simple fact of commerce.

Thousands of people go to McDonald's and enjoy a very affordable hamburger. It is easy to see that McDonald's would fall on their face if they tried to dress up their burger and charge five or six times as much for it. Common sense says that most people would wind up going to the grocery and then at home to fix a hamburger.

There is a tipping point in all commerce and business. Once the business person accepts that a Chevy will not bring the same price as a Cadillac and sells the Chevy at the Chevy's price, good things start to happen. When the chiropractic profession realizes they are trying to sell a Chevy at a Cadillac price changes can occur. If they start selling Chevy's at Chevy prices, good things will happen for everyone. Finally, the public will be able to get significant adjustments at a Chevy fee, and the chiropractors will also benefit when the masses start coming into their offices. When they start charging Chevy fees for Cadillac adjustments, you will bring all your friends and relatives to get adjusted. They will be overrun and may start complaining that they do not have time to go fishing. Wouldn't that be awesome! What a saintly thing for the chiropractors to do for you, to allow patients to beat a path to their doors to help you. Chiropractors then would succeed on the business side. They may not get to go fishing, but they could sing going to the office and the bank. Chiropractors need to know the location of the tipping point.

The Hundred-Year-Olds

I have been a chiropractor for over fifty years, and we have seen thousands of different people in our office and have the files to verify this information. In those files, you will find many people who we have taken care of that made it to ninety, ninety-five, and one-hundred-plus years. In my immediate family, I had an uncle who made it to one hundred. My father and mother made it to ninety-five, and my father-in-law to ninety-six. An aunt made it to ninety-eight. Three of my wife's cousins are still going, and all are over ninety years old. I've found that as patients age, their children begin moving them around for the child's connivance, and we lose track of them. However, in the ones that stayed with us, the thing that stood out most was that all of them had a straight spine.

Remember when I told you that you need to check your hips daily after you shower because you want your hips to be level? If they stay level, chances are you will remain in alignment and have pretty good health. For the fun of it, if you have an older parent in your family and they are doing well, check their hips. I will bet you a dollar to a donut that they will be level. Next, check someone who is not doing well. Again, I'll bet their hips will not be level.

Significantly, kids can have their teeth straightened, and it makes them look awesome. But isn't it sad that they may have subluxations, which go undetected for many years, causing myriads of conditions that could have been averted?

Let us go back to the hundred-year-olds. Somehow or some way they were lucky not to have any subluxations, vertebrae out of place, throughout their life. It could be luck. In my family and all my older patients, it was because they went to the chiropractor. They had their hips aligned, the sacral base leveled, and the spine straightened regularly or when they knew their hips were getting off-center.

You can go to a chiropractor who practices like we do in our office three or four times a year and spend less than you pay for a week's worth of groceries. Wow, am I saying you could live to be ninety to one hundred years old, be in good health until the day or week you pass away? And that you could do it for what a week's worth of groceries would cost each year? That is exactly what I am saying! Unbelievable? Not at all. Remember, you cannot wait till you are seventy to start this maintenance.

Life is like a stalk of corn; it is planted in May, shoots up all summer, then definitely after the first frost, the leaves and ear of corn start to turn down. We are the same way. For the first thirty-five years, we shoot up like the corn stalk, then at the age of thirty-five, we start to sag. You need to start your hip observation before age thirty-five. The country spends millions of dollars on cosmetic changes for straight teeth for our kids. Unfortunately, there is very little straightening of their spines. Spines are what will govern our health from childhood through the rest of our lives.

Ten-Year-Olds

The healthy future of any child relies on their hip balance and spinal structure—granted, they need a proper diet, exercise, rest, etc., which most parents address regularly. What is not discussed is structural alignment. The chiropractic profession should be ashamed for letting the public down by not giving them a method to stay healthy without pills.

A thirteen-year-old girl was in the office recently with a tale of woe. She was hit in the right temple with a softball, treated for a concussion, and developed devastating headaches and pain throughout her spine. Her doctor prescribed medications, ordered CT scans, MRIs, and X-rays, yet neck, midback, and low back pain persisted. Her grandmother could not stand her taking such powerful medications, all to no avail, and missing school with severe headaches. She brought her to us.

After a thorough history and chiropractic analysis, we determined that the first cervical vertebra had shifted to the left. The blow came from the right. It moved the skull to the left, much like a cup slipping on a saucer. We adjusted the first cervical vertebra, and she felt immediate relief. We made her stay and observed how she responded for twenty minutes, and she left feeling much better. She came back one week later for a checkup excited because she felt great. She exclaimed, "Dr. Ross, look at my hips. They have stayed level all week!" She went on to say that after leaving the office, they stopped at a mall two miles away. When she got out of the car, she knew she was okay.

Everyone is concerned about the dealer on the corner selling drugs to our children, but what does every medical doctor do? What example do we set? There are enough prescriptions written by medics for every man, woman, and child in America to have a dose of OxyContin every day for two and one half months. Monkey see monkey do! Chiropractors need to be teaching every parent how to check their kids' hips. Children do not need to grow into adulthood with the idea that good health comes from popping pills. They do not need to go into adulthood carrying subluxations that will create numerous conditions that will never be corrected. If children are adjusted and their spines kept straight in their growth years, could many disorders be prevented? I would say yes!

Currently, my profession is not interested in taking care of the ten-year-olds and teaching parents how to check their hips. Neither is my profession very interested in taking care of the hundred-year-old patients unless they have an excellent insurance plan. Of course, they would be on Medicare, and pay for chiropractic care is abysmal. Generally, it appears what chiropractors are interested in is how to get the most out of an insurance plan.

When you go to a chiropractor's office, you would expect that providing you with a beneficial adjustment would be foremost on their mind. Unfortunately, when you go into most chiropractor's offices, the most important thing on their mind is whether your insurance can pay. Will insurance cover fifteen adjustments, twenty-five physical therapy sessions, and thirty-five massages? Your health is secondary. There is no concern for the ten or hundred-year-olds.

Presently we are not interested in transforming ten-year-olds into healthy adults who can enjoy a healthy life for eight or nine more decades. Some studies say 70 percent of the population would consider utilizing chiropractic for structural care. People would love to have something other than pills for their health care. The chiropractic profession should feel guilty for not educating America's parents on this vitally important issue. Chiropractors, for their self-aggrandizement, want to be acceptable in the eyes of the elite. They know how to work the codes for a steady revenue stream, and for what? They see a whopping 5 percent of the population. Big deal. What if they started taking care of ten-year-olds and teaching parents how to check spines to help them flourish through life until they become hundred-year-olds? Now that is change.

Chiropractic has been treading water and standing still for so long that there is no excitement. Chiropractors say, "Come and get adjusted and you will feel healthy, happy, and terrific," which is true—you do feel much better. But the profession is going to have to change before we can improve the health of the world. Chiropractic can offer improved health to everyone, but it erects barriers, sits and spins its wheels going nowhere. Chiropractic needs to grow, tear down the barricades, and see 95 percent of the population not for the benefit of chiropractors but for the sake of humanity!

CHAPTER 35

Deep Pockets

Chiropractors are the only health care providers who can give the medics competition and lower health costs. It would be easy to provide them with competition by seeing more patients. If patients were flowing into chiropractor's offices, they wouldn't need to compete with the medics for money from the insurance well. At some point, chiropractors need to realize that insurance money is the medics' money. They are no different than a dog with a bone. Do dogs have morals? Do dogs think they have to share with another dog? No, when another dog tries to steal their bone, there is going to be gnashing of teeth. Chiropractors should focus on getting paid from the patient in smaller amounts for their intangible adjustment. Patients will love to pay when you produce at a reasonable fee they can afford, especially when they receive great benefits.

Insurance and Dishonesty: Is It Worth It?

Sadly, the pitiful chiropractors accept the leftovers of insurance handouts and keep trying to tap into that cache. Chiropractors took an oath that says they are to be honest with their patients. All chiropractors, along with all healthcare providers, know insurance can easily make you dishonest. We do not utilize insurance in our office because of the dishonesty factor. It is easy to add whatever you want to an insurance form. There are many X-rays taken and charged for but never read.

A chiropractor told me years ago that he x-rayed most of his patients and had his unit rigged in a way that the motor ran but would not take an X-ray. When the time came to show the patient their films, he had two or three developed X-rays that he would rotate and display for the patient. He would tell the patient it was theirs and charge them the full fee for an X-ray series. He pulled this trick for years, got away with it, and was never confronted with the scam.

My wife's mother was hospitalized three days before her death. The doctor making rounds charged $150 on two different occasions for looking at her chart for five seconds. The chart was behind a screen, and he never once looked at the patient on those two visits.

Insurance has deep pockets. Essentially it is socialism—everyone pools their money, and doctors get to use the pooled money for the sickest 20 percent of the population. These two groups are the only ones who benefit from the hard-earned money contributed to the pool. Socialism destroys character and alters ideals. Chiropractors took an oath to help the public, not to fleece them. Chiropractors argue that the medics do it. Yes, but does that make it right? Do we, as a profession, have to act like the medics? Ever since Medicare came into being, we have been sitting on the back row waiting to lap up leftover insurance money. The result is that the profession sees little of the population. That is a shame because it deprives millions of people of experiencing the benefit of a beneficial chiropractic adjustment.

Chiropractors will never get to use insurance like the medics. Should we want to because of the dishonesty? Today, tests medics perform and receive compensation for provide more information that they need to pursue. A school-teacher patient who came periodically for an adjustment was retiring at the end of the school year. He told me he was going in for a physical exam to make sure everything was okay before retirement. I did not see him for over a year, and when I did, he had a horror story to relate. When he had his medical exam, everything was essentially normal except for the PSA test. It was way too high for a healthy prostate. They checked the prostate several times, and it still registered high. In light of the testing results, it was determined that prostate surgery was necessary for urine to pass more efficiently. Unfortunately, he had the operation, and it left him wearing a diaper. Until this physical, which led to testing and then to an invasive procedure, this man was a healthy, robust individual. It is truly a sad situation. Tests find conditions that sometimes it's better not to see. Many times, God can take care of these things better than man. Sadly in reality, this all happened because he had "good insurance." Do we, as chiropractors, want to find some of these conditions when it may be better just to let them run their course?

We should concentrate on helping everyone by giving effective adjustments that are affordable. Allowing patients to pay cash and not fight over the same 5 percent of the population that already goes to chiropractors would help everyone. If we opened our doors in this manner, the world would beat a path to our door.

Insurance is for catastrophic problems. Vertebra being out of place causing spinal misalignment can be life-changing, but it hardly equates to catastrophic. Devastation and catastrophes occur. Does the chiropractic profession want to spend its time in this arena? It is not its expertise. Is it worth spending time trying to wrestle crumbs from the medics insurance cache? We could be seeing a high percentage of the population, having fun, and receiving accolades for a job well done? We do have acres of diamonds in our backyard.

We all know someone who has had a knee replacement. Using a stationary bike on a regular basis may keep your knees working longer.

KNEES

One of the best methods to save your knees is to ride a stationary bike 10 minutes before going to bed.

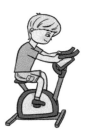

All day long your activity and weight compresses your knee joints.

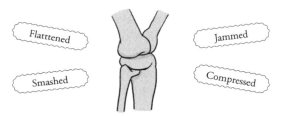

By riding leisurely, with no tension on the wheel, this activity pries open and frees the compression and jamming.

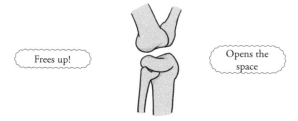

If you will go straight to bed, this space will remain open. This will allow extra blood to irrigate the area and help with tissue and cartilage repair.

The Fifth Reformation—
Education

CHAPTER 36

Addiction

At this moment in time, chiropractic students are spending an excessive amount of time learning insurance billing and coding and precious little time learning how to detect and correct hips, sacrum, and spines. Throughout this book, I have been pretty hard on my fellow chiropractors. I'm trying to make them feel guilty as hell for not taking care of 95 percent of the people rather than the 5 percent who will pay them with insurance. Analogous to Nero, who fiddled while Rome burned, many chiropractors feel to heck with the 95 percent, "I'll take my easy insurance money." The profession turns a blind eye to all your suffering and forces you to run to the medic for pain pills. When in reality, a couple of adjustments would get you back to work.

Chiropractors' fiddling while the majority of the population goes without the opportunity to be adjusted is caused by the misguided mission and goals of our chiropractic colleges. Today chiropractic students are not taught how to use one of the greatest gifts anyone could receive. This gift is the ability to make God's children feel healthy and functional by using only their hands and the skills taught to them. Chiropractic translates from Latin to mean "with hands only." Our schools should be concentrating on adjusting skills versus billing and coding. Perhaps one day the educational authorities of my profession will quit isolating themselves from mainline education and let curriculum directors from our top universities help them. Maybe then we will have a doctoral program geared to helping the masses instead of those few that have proper insurance.

Presently our schools are teaching a format set up when chiropractic started its first school in 1904. It has never changed; all that has occurred is adding medical courses on top of more medical courses. It is time for the profession to come out of the nineteenth century and quit isolating our educational programs. We act like we have something to hide by not asking general education professionals to look at what we are doing. We are not using the wealth of mainstream colleges and universities. There is a plethora of experts who could assist in organizing and structuring chiropractic's educational curriculum.

The educational setup is the culprit. The current system is trying to do two things at one time. On the one hand, it wants its graduates to be doctors. A doctoral program aims to concentrate on the candidate becoming an authority in one field. This is the format used by all educational institutions except the chiropractic profession. Chiropractic schools profess that they want their graduates to be doctors who are more or less isolated into one field, much like a specialist. A specialist is one who knows more and more about less and less.

On the other hand, they wind up doing the exact opposite of the accepted doctoral format. More and more medical courses and fields of endeavor are offered. They are like the Olympics, which each year adds more sports to their venue, or a restaurant that continually adds more dishes to their menu. Pretty soon, it is overwhelming, and you do not know what game to watch or what meal to try.

Watering It Down

Chiropractic always has and still is diversifying, and this diversification leads to a watering down of its primary philosophy. By watering down, I mean it makes you know less and less about more and more. The chiropractic doctorate is a dichotomy. It wants branding, but it is more interested in being all things to everyone for everything.

Our profession loves to point out that we have more educational hours than medical doctors at Johns Hopkins University. Even so, the profession has mired itself in the nineteenth and twentieth century's educational formats while trying to add some twenty-first-century medical courses and insurance codes to make it look acceptable. They spend much time and effort trying to be a medic and finding that elusive key to the insurance lockbox. In their greed for the almighty dollar and acceptance, they have forgotten their reason for going into chiropractic. Most of us went into the profession to help people, all people, regardless of color, creed, or financial ability to pay. Perhaps we should add, "or insurance affiliation." In the end, all these so-called educational improvements have done is to water down chiropractic and make it unavailable to 95 percent of the population. A great accomplishment for 125 years of service!

Jack of All Trades

Chiropractic has been expanding its doctoral degree program more and more into every health care field except drugs, dentistry, and surgery. It teaches doctors to be diverse, to expand into more areas, which is the opposite of what the doctoral degree is all about. Earlier, we referred to the Carnegie Report, which described why doctorates were set up as they are as a means to protect the public. The developers of the educational procedures did not want a specialist doing all sorts of ventures because they then become a jack of all trades and master of none. The chiropractic profession finds itself in this position today, the proverbial Jack of all trades. Do you see why the friend in Chicago got hoodwinked by the so-called chiropractor who turned out to be a chiropractic physician who was Dr. Jack of All Trades? Instead of obtaining the adjustment she wanted, he sold her a bill of goods she did not wish to receive.

When you go to a medical doctor, a dentist, or a podiatrist, you know what you are going to receive. They are not going to hustle you into things outside of their expertise. They will not try to convince you that you need fire cupping, GuaSha, smoking cessation, weight reduction, cosmetic acupuncture, or any other of the many modalities found in chiropractor's offices today. No, they are professionals working within their doctoral program limitations. They are not hustlers. Specializing allows quality control. You want to go to a dentist who knows how to drill and has become an expert at drilling. Does drilling and more drill-ing become tiresome? It possibly does. For the medic, I presume sitting across a desk and writing script for one patient after another could get boring. But that is what doctorates and specializing are all about.

Herein lies the chiropractic problem: its doctorate program teaches more and more about more and more. This procedure is the opposite of what the rest of the world's doctoral programs teach. As I write this, several state chiropractic associations are clamoring for rights to prescriptive drugs. They use the osteopathic profession as an exam-ple. Osteopathic doctors have increased their numbers by incorporat-ing prescriptive drugs. (Note: Osteopaths started out manipulating the spine and then went to drug therapy. Today, a few osteopaths will manipulate but only when all else fails.)

Several years ago, I had been taking care of a seventy-year-old man with left leg sciatica. At that time, I was in the office on Saturday. A younger man came in and said that he was my patient's son and wanted to discuss his father's progress. He introduced himself as being from Grand Rapids and was spending the weekend with his father. He said he was an osteopath and asked to see his father's X-rays.

We consented and showed him the films. His dad had a prob-lem with the alignment of his left hip and, with our care, was improv-ing nicely. We discussed his father's case. As he was leaving, he said to me, "You chiropractors are nuts to do all that heavy physical work of adjusting patients. You need to get prescription rights as we have. It is so much easier." He went on to say, "In my dad's case, as good as his X-rays looked, I would have given him pain pills laced with a muscle relaxer. I would never have had to do anything but push the envelope." He then added, "Before I came over here this afternoon, I stopped at the hospital and stuck my head in on seven patients. Just for just ducking in and out, I collected seventy-five dollars for each visit." He was deadly serious! Wow, no wonder the state associations want to move into the main-stream of health care and be able to write all those opioid prescriptions.

First of all, if chiropractors would get drug rights, they would be like the osteopaths. Soon the chiropractor would not be adjusting at all because of the physical work involved. Secondly, why would they want to drug this world any more than it already is? Would this not be a moral issue?

Typically, the people who promote this type of thinking within the profession never wanted to be a chiropractor in the first place. They are the ones who could not get into medical school and entered the chiropractic field just to become a doctor. Now they want to make chiropractic acceptable to themselves. These are the same people who push for more and more medical education, which they think will make them more accepted. They have been diversifying the profession for many years, and it now takes additional years to get through chiropractic school.

Presently, at the National College of Chiropractic (now called the National University of Health Sciences) in Lombard, Illinois, it takes nine years from high school to receive a doctoral degree. They have a bachelor's degree requirement for entrance, but many of the profession's schools will allow acceptance with two years of college. With only a two-year requirement, you can complete your chiropractic degree in seven years. Mostly the degrees from the various schools are the same. There is a lot of leeway in laws governing the practice of chiropractic in each state. These laws allow chiropractors to administer a myriad of health care modalities, many of which they did not study in school. There is a disconnect between schools with no absolute standardization of education or an emphasis on specialization. It becomes a quagmire of more and more diversification. The result is more and more seat time in the classroom, leading to more debt as the graduates leave school. Unfortunately, they graduate without having a game plan as to the most efficient process in taking care of patients.

Much like the child with too many toys, the new graduate is not entirely competent in any one specialty. They become frustrated because they cannot zero in on how best to manage a patient. The result is poor patient management, which causes inadequate patient response leading to reduced income, which leads to the inability to pay off the enormous tuition debt. These responses are leading reasons almost 50 percent of all chiropractic graduates fail after five years in practice. What a catastrophe. This failure rate after five years is terrible. It is mainly because our school's doctoral program is teaching our candidates to be diversified instead of zeroing in on the adjustment. It is the opposite of the accepted standard doctoral program recognized in all mainstream colleges and universities. We are producing a jack of all trades and calling them a doctor. I believe they call this an oxymoron!

Tarred and Feathered

Fifty percent of all graduates fail after five years? Our chiropractic school authorities should be scalded, tarred, and feathered. It is deplorable to allow students to amass $250,000 in tuition debt and not provide a clear-cut avenue for them to pay back their obligation. Not to mention, they graduate without a game plan to help the patients who put their trust in the new practitioner for their care. How are 50 percent of our graduates failing after five years in practice when 95 percent of the population is starving for an adjustment? So many diamonds in our backyard, yet we cannot see them.

Adam Smith, the great economist of the seventeenth century, observed that when specialization took place, it far outweighed diversification, and good things happened for all. Adam Smith noted four hundred years ago that the diversification the state associations want is outdated. To all you progressive chiropractors who are still living in the eighteenth century of diversification, this is not progression; it is regression!

These wannabe medics just do not get it. They are obsessed with the self-aggrandizement of being a medic. They add more and more medical courses to our curriculum. Additional courses will restrict students from entering school due to lengthening the time necessary to graduate, thus, leading to more failures for the students who do come.

To my knowledge, no one in the hierarchy of the profession has addressed the educational problem from a common-sense approach. They have never requested institutions of higher learning to show chiropractic the proper formats and curriculums that mainline university doctoral programs utilize.

Eventually, the profession will have to allow the educational experts from the university to come and advise them if the profession is to grow and thrive. There are curriculum directors in every state university system who would be more than happy to offer their expertise. To produce a curriculum that would enable the chiropractic profession to pull itself out of the eighteenth-century educational system would be a challenge. Introducing a twenty-first century doctoral program for chiropractic to make it a viable and productive profession is a necessity.

Like any addict, chiropractic has to realize they have a problem before they can accept help. Authorities in my profession want to add drugs to their addiction. If they get their way, say goodbye to affordable adjustments.

CHAPTER 37

The Stockholm Syndrome

In the profession's unrelenting quest to become more medically oriented, I liken the plight of the chiropractors to the hostages in the famous and notorious Stockholm syndrome case.

In 1973, bank robbers in Stockholm, Sweden, took four hostages during their robbery spree. The captives made a valiant effort to build an alliance with the robbers as a survival strategy. Does this sound familiar? Chiropractors have been desperately trying to develop an alliance with the medics ever since they set out to destroy the chiropractors in the 1920s and '30s.

The Carnegie Foundation, along with the medics and the help of the federal government, went after the chiropractors attempting to annihilate these upstarts and what they called the poor boys from the health care system. By 1920, there were thirty thousand practicing chiropractors in the field. People were getting great results, and chiropractic was sweeping across the country like a wildfire.

The medics, feeling the heat, decided to stop this scorching of the health care field. The method that would eliminate these upstarts was the formation of state licensing boards.

Licensing boards were set up in every state, and of course, medics and dentists were the only ones licensed. Anyone else hanging out a shingle was practicing medicine without a license. They were arrested, jailed, fined, and asked to leave town.

This blitzkrieg started in the early 1920s with thirty thousand chiropractors on the roles. By the 1930s, the number had been reduced to five thousand or less. Most chiropractors scuttled the ship, but the strongest and most determined stayed aboard. Many of them paid a hefty price for chiropractic. For example, Dr. Frank Reeves, who practiced in Cincinnati, went to jail twenty-nine times for the cause. The strong ones like him were not going to let the government and medics annihilate them.

Therefore, like the Stockholm hostages trying to plot a survival plan with their captors, the chiropractors had to figure out a survival approach that would keep the profession afloat. The logical way would be to obtain a license. Licensure did eventually become the answer to the chiropractor's protection. It came with a high price, not so much for the chiropractors but you the public.

The job of the chiropractor is to adjust the spine. That is what state governments licensed chiropractors to do. The adjustment of the spine is the vehicle that allows chiropractic to exist. Was it dumb luck, a foreseeable plan by the medics, or sheer stupidity on the part of chiropractors? Almost every state now allows chiropractors the ability to practice any holistic therapy ever conceived under the chiropractic law. Consequently, chiropractors have developed an alliance with some medical/insurance companies to dispense some of their monies on holistic care.

Placing multitudinous therapies under the chiropractic license umbrella, it has made the chiropractor a jack of all trades and master of none. What is the result of allowing the chiropractor to be so diversified? You guessed it. It keeps chiropractors occupied with therapies and trying to get paid for them. They do not have time to give all of you an amazing affordable adjustment, which you need so badly.

The medics could not do away with chiropractors in the 1930s, and they had to go along with licensing them because it is so effective that the public demanded it. The medics had an invisible hand in helping water down the real practice of chiropractic, which is adjusting the spine only. The act of adjusting the spine is what scares the pants off the medics. By keeping the chiropractors running therapy machines, they are not adjusting spines and getting people well. Therapy machines keep chiropractors spinning their wheels, which is what the medics want.

By running these machines and begging for insurance money to pay for these therapies, we are effectively hostages of the medics. It continues to this day. In the spring of 2018, the Indiana General Assembly passed a bill allowing chiropractors to "dry needle" their patients, which is somehow different than acupuncture, which is not permitted. I attended a seminar shortly after its passage for my annual license renewal credit hours. The instructor was teaching dry needling. It is somewhat like acupuncture, yet after ten hours of lecture, I'm still not sure what it is suitable for or how it should be utilized. Curiously, this presenter was more excited that insurance companies will pay for this service and emphasized over and over not to screw up the codes because they will pay well for this service.

Insurance paying for dry needling is just another illustration of how the profession is obsessed with being allied to the medics and medical insurance. Jumping up and down, falling all over themselves when their medical captors are friendly to them is amusing, instead of doing the right thing, telling the medics to buzz off. Our job is to start doing what we should be doing, adjusting everyone in the world. Nevertheless, we keep playing with therapies. The profession cannot shake free of their captors, the medics. They are afraid. Like the Stockholm hostages, they do not want to offend their captors because they may not give them any more goodies. Similar to the Stockholm case, it was not about justice, but rather themselves, the hostages.

My seminar teacher was mostly interested in whether the chiropractors could get paid. But what about helping the public? The world is being robbed of life-saving adjustments all because the profession is obsessed with the medics and insurance payments. This hostage mentality has existed for the last eighty years and has to cease. The profession needs to grow up and stand on its own two feet not for the profession's sake but for all suffering people in the world that chiropractors could help immensely.

CHAPTER 38

History and Wannabees

There is a specific reason my profession is full of wannabees. It stems directly from our history. To understand this plight, I will take you through part of our colorful history. As we have said before, nothing is written in the media about chiropractic. It is a faceless profession. It leaves no scars, and it doesn't see a tremendous number of people. In the early days of the profession, BJ Palmer, the developer of chiropractic, wrote thirty-nine books on chiropractic. Most of these books are out of print, and it is hard to find copies. The reason for archiving these books is because they are an embarrassment to the wannabees. Someday they will come out of hiding because Palmer was way ahead of his time. Naturally, he made mistakes—one of which I will take him to task. His educational format and the way he prepared students to face the world was adequate for the time. But it needs to be drastically changed if chiropractic is going to make a worldwide impact.

Chiropractic was founded in 1895 by DD Palmer. He was not excited about starting a school to train people to become chiropractors. His son, BJ, was adamant that a school should be initiated to spread this good news of how chiropractic could and should help restore and maintain health. BJ eventually developed a school based on the adjustment of subluxated vertebrae. He demonstrated that the correction of subluxated vertebrae would ease patients' pain and suffering.

He had no scientific proof that his distracters wanted, but he had testimonials. When people feel better, they really could care less about scientific evidence. Therefore, with all the positive feedback they were getting from correcting subluxations, he did not listen to critics. He persevered and continued teaching that the job of the chiropractor was to reset or adjust the subluxated vertebra.

Unfortunately, diversification began the very first year that the Palmer School was in existence because BJ had one of the first wannabees as a student. From the very beginning, chiropractic had its detractors. This student of BJ's was a so-called medical doctor who practiced water therapy, which was the practice of dripping water onto a lesion for healing purposes. This student did not think chiropractic should stand alone as a separate healing art or entity. He believed BJ's philosophy and teachings were that chiropractic was a cure-all for all conditions and diseases, and he thought this was absurd. BJ did say that subluxations were the cause of disease but not necessarily all disease. However, he later amended it to a subluxation was the cause of *dis-ease*. As chiropractors, we correct subluxations that take the pressure off a malpositioned vertebra, which allows the nervous system to help relieve the dis-ease that existed in the body. Subluxations do alter body function and cause the body to be ill-at-ease.

The student mentioned above that disagreed with BJ was John Fitz Howard, who, in his early thirties, was some fifteen years older than BJ. Howard was upset that DD Palmer, BJ's father, was not teaching the courses. Howard wanted the old man that founded chiropractic but instead was lectured by this snot-nosed kid who acted as though he was the world's authority on chiropractic. He did not like the young kid teaching him. He stated many times that he knew more about chiropractic than this youngster, and he would be a much better teacher of the subject than BJ.

Howard never thought that chiropractic was a stand-alone therapy. He felt that it should be used in conjunction with other therapies and should be one of the many tools he kept in his black bag. This was the thinking of the first wannabe, Dr. John Howard, 120-plus years ago and is still the thinking of today's wannabees. These chiropractors cannot or will not accept the premise that the body is a structure that has to be in alignment for it to function efficiently. Anything you can think of—machines, doors, windows—all work best when they are in alignment.

Structure was not paramount in Dr. Howard's thinking, and he could not conceive the importance that it plays in overall health as the Palmers envisioned. Alteration of the body from outside forces was the mindset of Howard, the wannabees, medical doctors, and society as a whole. With today's advertisements touting how miraculous drugs are for curing everything, people go to the medic demanding what they saw on TV. Their medic gets out the prescription pad and introduces the patient to the drug world or enables those who have already started down the drug's path. Anyone going into a medical doctor's office today will usually not exit without a prescription slip. Medics do not have to work at pushing drugs; the drug company advertisements do it for them. This gold mine the medics have is the envy of all wannabe chiropractors, and they salivate wanting to get on that gravy train. Just how much money is being made by the medics pushing all these drugs? Check out the top fifty stocks on the New York Stock Exchange, a high percentage of them are drug or healthcare related.

If Dr. John Could Have Foreseen

If Dr. John Howard could have foreseen the vast role drugs would play in the medical profession, he probably would never have trifled with chiropractic. At that time, drugs, as we have today, were not around. If they had been, chances are he would have put them in his black bag instead of adding chiropractic as one of his treatments. Possibly this would have been a blessing for all of us.

He thought BJ was nuts for saying that chiropractic could stand alone and for not believing that chiropractic needed complementary treatments to get a person well. Therefore, after sitting in BJ's class for four months, Howard had all he could take and walked out. He did not go far, just down the hill toward the river on Brady Street in Davenport and started a school of his own.

He named his school the National College of Chiropractic but did not stay long on Brady Street. Because of his medical leanings, he wanted to be near a medical facility, so he moved it to Chicago to be close to the Rush Medical School. For many years, he was able to have his chiropractic students reciprocate with the medical school. Eventually, his school moved to the suburb of Lombard, Illinois, where it exists today.

Dr. Howard started his school in 1904 and, with his medical leanings, divided the profession then. National keeps it divided to this day. The school has changed its name to the National University of Health Sciences. It continues to promote its progressive movement by trying to incorporate drugs, oriental medicine, acupuncture, physical therapy, and massage and call their graduates doctors of chiropractic medicine. They teach diversity, yet the chiropractic adjustment is the only thing licensed and sanctioned that gives National the right to exist as an institution.

National says, even though the subluxation is the essence of chiropractic and upon what the laws exist, it has never been proven. Thus, subluxations do not exist. They go on to say our belief in this subluxation, which cannot be verified, is why the scientific world will not accept us, and this is an embarrassment to the wannabees. Dr. Howard and his National offspring have the right to practice because of the subluxation theory. They do not like what it stands for, but they exploit it for their agenda.

Chiropractic came into being in 1895 to structurally maintain spines, thereby giving people a better opportunity to live longer and healthier lives. However, Dr. Howard believed it to be just another therapy that belonged in his black bag to use as an adjunct when nothing else worked.

Notice the difference. We will use it once in a while when we feel it will fit in with our treatment protocol per Howard or BJ's concept that everyone should have the right and opportunity to have their spine adjusted as necessary.

Howard could not accept BJ's belief that the chiropractor needed to stick to analyzing the spine, locating and correcting subluxations. BJ said everyone on the planet has a spine, and it needs to be aligned periodically. Everybody should have the opportunity to be adjusted for their body to function optimally, which reduces the risk of dis-ease and, ultimately, disease.

Medicine treats people's symptoms with pills, ointments, and injections, which mask the problems. Many of the causes of missed workdays are structural problems. Adjustments can get most patients back on the job in a day or two. So why do the wannabe chiropractors want to treat patients with a pill that is just a cover-up when so many people need to get back on the job as quickly as possible?

Can you see the contrast in vision between our two early leaders of chiropractic? Palmer's philosophy was to make the world healthy by keeping spines straight, while Howard's was to treat sore throats. There was a difference in their visions, and those differences exist today.

BJ opened his school in 1904 at the age of nineteen and held steadfast to his philosophy, and the Palmer School became a success. By 1920, thirty thousand chiropractors had graduated, and the vast majority were adjusting spines like crazy throughout the United States. By doing such a good job, they were projected into the spotlight of the medics and their cohorts in the government, and that spelled trouble.

CHAPTER 39

BJ, the Wonder Kid and the Little Red Engine

From the age of nineteen to the age of thirty-nine, BJ developed into one of America's foremost geniuses and entrepreneurs. In his heyday, he paralleled Thomas Edison, John Deere, and Henry Ford and, in many ways, had a considerable effect on the American public. If he had not had the competition of the government and medical profession, straight chiropractors would be seeing 95 percent of the population today. The name Palmer would rank along with Ford and Deere. But the government and the medics did everything in their power to impede his progress and shut him down. He was able to defeat this attempted destruction, but they did eventually slow down the Palmer impetus that produced the thirty thousand chiropractors who were taking the country by storm in the 1920s. Since they could not stop him, because his principle was right, the government and medics had to give in and compromise. They gave in by forcing us to be similar to them so they could control us via licensure.

The government eventually issued licenses in every state based on a compromise. Chiropractic could exist on Palmer's subluxation basis. But chiropractors would have to make a medical diagnosis to prove there is a subluxation. Palmer said we analyze the spine; we do not diagnose. If one does diagnose, it leads to a medical decision, and a medical condition is not treated with an adjustment. No medical textbook in the country states an adjustment is a preferred treatment for a medical condition. Analysis and diagnosis are two different things, and they are antithetical.

To become licensed, the profession had to accept this dichotomy. Regrettably, the need to make a medical diagnosis plays into the hands of the wannabees. They get to make a medical diagnosis, then treat it with a conjured treatment that sort of parallels what the medical textbook describes for that diagnosis. Because of the diagnosis, they no longer have to treat it with an adjustment. They can use nutrition, physical therapy, acupuncture, laser, massage, weight reduction, smoking cessation, and on and on. Chiropractic exists and holds the license to practice entirely via the subluxation. Insurance doesn't pay well for a subluxation because it is unscientific. However, it pays the chiropractor well for all the things that are not chiropractic and for which they do not have a license for. That was the compromise. The medics and the government knew what they were doing by making the chiropractors a jack of all trades. It keeps them diversified, busy trying to get crumbs from the insurance companies, and in so doing, they will not be competition. It appears, after all these years, with the chiropractic profession only seeing 5 percent of the population, it is working pretty darned well.

Today the Little Red Engine of chiropractic chugs along pulling about ten cars. Each one is full of nutrition, physical therapy, acupuncture, exercise therapy, laser therapy, workout gyms for muscle building therapy, medical massage therapy, wellness therapy, weight reduction therapy, or pain management therapy. More cars continue to be added. Now Dr. Howard's school, National, wants to add drug therapy. The Little Red Engine has a massive load and is presently overloaded by all these therapies. The wannabees would eliminate chiropractic if it were not for BJ and the Little Red Engine that carries them along with the license to practice in the first place.

CHAPTER 40

The Government and Medics Are Winning

While the government and medics are winning, the public is losing! Although the chiropractic profession accepts what the government and medics have dealt them, they have tried for the last one hundred years to blend the two aspects of the professions. We see such a small percentage of the population that it is not working. It will never work!

It is a terrible shame that the leaders of my profession cannot see the problem, because chiropractors are letting masses of you suffer needlessly. The biblical parable of hiding the talents in a hole sure fits our profession.

Can this be remedied? It sure can. It can be readily corrected; all we need to do is to get some egos out of the way. Once that is accomplished, chiropractic can help reduce and control health care costs plus make everyone feel better once they have access to a chiropractor who will adjust the spine. The physical aspect of educating chiropractors is minor, which I will show you shortly. Overcoming the ego factor becomes the most significant difficulty.

CHAPTER 41

First-Hand Experience

I have had a BJ Palmer/John Howard experience of my own. Due to this experience, I know that if common sense and utilization of the universal educational system of producing doctoral candidates would ever prevail, the chiropractic profession would be able to open their doors, allowing everyone to get adjusted. BJ Palmer and John Howard began together in 1904. Both were chiropractors, but each went in opposite directions.

In 1964, I entered the National College of Chiropractic that Dr. John Howard started sixty years earlier. In my class was a fellow by the name of Jim Winterstein. For the next four years, we sat together in every class and studied chiropractic. Most chiropractic schools are small, and my school had approximately three hundred students, with forty-three students in my class. In chiropractic school, you stay with the same group until you graduate. It is not like the university where all your friends are pursuing different courses of study. All the chiropractic courses are taken in the same order. We study the same material, and our end goal is the same.

Chiropractic now has national and international schools. It began in Davenport, Iowa, and is as American as apple pie. There are fifteen chiropractic schools in this country, with a few overseas.

In my class, there were eleven international students. The American students were from all over the United States. Interestingly, I was the only one from Indiana. Chiropractic schools are unique in the fact that they are a melting pot, where people from all over the world come together and learn how to adjust, align hips, level sacrums, and straighten spines. Chiropractic adjustments can be given to anyone regardless of their ability to communicate, their political persuasion, or their religion. Once the art has been learned, all the chiropractor has to have is their hands to give an adjustment. No other health care professionals can do that. This unique phenomenon draws students from all over the world to study chiropractic.

The five-year curriculum is intense. We are in class for six hours per day, five days a week. Compare those hours to the university format, where you carry an average of sixteen hours per week. That is sixteen hours versus thirty hours for chiropractic school. Thirty hours is a challenging load. When I went to school, it was eight semesters in length, and now it has been extended to ten semesters.

I had graduated from Ball State Teachers College two years prior and taught elementary school before entering National in 1964. Ball State, at that time, was the top-ranked teacher's college in the Midwest. Professors were strict, and courses were designed to be tough and geared to flunk students who could not meet high standards. They strived for a high-attrition rate because they did not want teachers who did not have the proper grasp of the English language and subject matter. Therefore, I had a benchmark to compare National's instructors to some of the Midwest's best professors. I was very pleased with the majority of National's professors. We had a technique instructor, Dr. Alfred States, who was exceptionally well organized for class every day and was able to keep us busy from bell to bell. He taught and inspired us to become the best spinal adjustors possible. I could not have asked for a more organized, dedicated, demanding, knowledgeable, and passionate instructor. Out of the fifteen or more teachers we had at National, there were only three that were barely adequate.

All forty-three classmates got to know one another quite well. When you are together in the same setting for six hours daily, five days a week for four or more years, you become well acquainted. We absorbed what National had to offer concerning the basics and principles of chiropractic. My friend Jim Winterstein and I sat in every class listening, studying, and digesting the premise of chiropractic. Jim was brilliant.

He could read something once, and the picture would stick or listen to something one time and have it memorized. Jim was one of those fellows that you knew would be a leader and make a name for himself.

Jim had a warm personality; even with his intellectual gifts, he did not alienate anyone. We all liked Jim. He and I became good friends and still are to this day. Therefore, anything I say from this point forward has nothing to do with my friendship with Jim. Our relationship is excellent, but I will use it to explain why there is a division between the straight chiropractors and the medically oriented chiropractors. I will tell why there is no growth in the profession and why we only see 5 percent of the population. Once you have perused our relationship and understand that this environment is prevalent in every chiropractic school, then we can all better understand that chiropractic has some monumental problems.

The four years passed, and we all went our separate ways. Jim had a private practice for a while, then he moved into X-ray technology. Eventually, this interest led him back to National, where he taught and did research in the X-ray technology department. Jim was so astute in his subject that roughly seventeen years postgraduation, he was named the president of National, a position which he held for twenty-eight years until retiring in 2013.

I was delighted that one of my friends was appointed the president of our school. Not many graduates from National can boast that one of their classmates became president. Since its inception in 1904, they have had only four (there were some interims) permanent presidents, and only one of those four was a graduate of National. When one of your friends does well, it is very gratifying. While Jim was president, I attended National for license renewal and homecomings two or three times per year. I would joke with friends that I was one of the few people that could park in the president's reserved space or prop my feet on his desk and get by with it. It was a fun time.

CHAPTER 42

We Go Our Separate Ways

It was exciting to go back to homecomings, where all our classmates would tell the same old tales and lies of our school days. When we were in school, our president, Dr. Joseph Janse loved to quote from Rudyard Kipling's poem "The Stranger," especially the fourth stanza:

> The Stranger within my gate,
> He may be true or kind,
> But he does not talk my talk—
> I cannot feel his mind.
> I see the face and the eyes and the mouth,
> But not the soul behind.
>
> The men of my own stock,
> They may do ill or well,
> But they tell the lies I am wanted to,
> They are used to the lies I tell:
> And we do not need interpreters
> When we go to buy or sell.
>
> The Stranger within my gates,
> He may be evil or good,
> But I cannot tell what powers control—
> What reasons sway his mood;

Nor when the Gods of his far-off land
Shall repossess his blood

The men of my own stock,
Bitter bad they may be,
But, at least, they hear the things I hear,
And see the things I see;
And whatever I think of them and their likes
They think of the likes of me.

This was my father's belief
And this is also mine:
Let the corn be all one sheaf—
And the grapes be all one vine,
Ere our children's teeth are set on edge
By bitter bread and wine.

When we return for alumni gatherings, we do not discuss the split of chiropractic; we talk of our days in school and all the crazy pranks and shenanigans we pulled. Once we left school, we went in different directions to practice a myriad of ways.

John Howard walked out of BJ Palmer's College of Straight Chiropractic, went down the street, and started the first mixing school of chiropractic. In 1968, my class graduated and left National. Half went the Howard way, and the other half practiced some version of the Palmer straight method. Today in 2020, the profession is still split after 116 years.

Dr. Jim became a mixer. In chiropractic circles, a mixer is one who uses all sorts of holistic therapies and medical devices on their patients. Like Dr. Howard, they view chiropractic as something they want to keep in their black bag and use for specific conditions. They chose the medical-oriented path. On the other hand, like Robert Frost's poem "The Road Not Taken," I took the path less traveled, the straight chiropractic road. My friend Jim liked diagnosing, and I liked adjusting.

Because of the educational diversity and choices presented to us, our roads diverged. He took the more worn medical/diagnostic road, and I took the grassy, less-traveled one of aligning hips, leveling sacrums, and adjusting the spine. Thus, we went our separate ways professionally.

CHAPTER 43

Over Fifty Years of Adjusting

In the past fifty-two years, all I have done is adjust patients by aligning hips, leveling sacrums, and correcting subluxations. As I have mentioned, between my wife, my brother-in-law (they are brother and sister chiropractors), and myself, we have seen over 150,000 new patients and have administered over 1.5 million patient visits in the office. Our location is in the middle of northern Indiana, known as the Michiana area. The communities of Niles and Edwardsburg, Michigan, South Bend, Mishawaka, Elkhart, Jimtown, Osceola, Dunlap, and Goshen, Indiana, make up a population of over half a million people. That means our office has roughly seen over 30 percent of the community.

There were seven chiropractors in the area when we opened in 1975, and today we boast of having over seventy-five practicing chiropractors. Our office will see forty to sixty new patients per week, where 80 percent will get great results from one to three visits. They get very excited about their outcomes and tell friends and relatives. Down the road, when a need arises, those friends and relatives come to the office. People love to come. They like the results, but due to the demand for our services, the line gets quite long and the wait time can take two or three hours. With such an overflow of patients, our area became fertile ground for young chiropractors to set up a practice on our doorstep. Many young chiropractors opened offices close by, and that is the reason we now have seventy-five chiropractors in our area.

What is tremendous about this story is it has come about through word of mouth. We have never advertised, and you will see very few of the other seventy-five chiropractors advertising, except for one high roller. The national average indicates that chiropractors only see 5 percent of the population. Our office alone has seen 30 percent in our area. Factor in all the other seventy-plus chiropractors in our area that seem to be doing well, and I will venture to say that chiropractors in our area may be seeing close to 50 percent of our population.

Let us go back to Dr. Jim and me graduating from the same school and becoming two different animals. Dr. Jim changed the name of the National College of Chiropractic to the National University of Health Sciences while he was president. Here he taught students to be chiropractic physicians who want to be all things to their patients. By giving a condition a medical diagnosis, then trying to treat that condition with a therapy they think would parallel what the medic would perform becomes their objective. The school qualifies as a university by adding a massage school, where you can learn to be a masseuse. They also added physiotherapy, acupuncture, and oriental medicine schools. The title of doctor of chiropractic became a doctor of chiropractic medicine. *Medicine* was included in the title because they are hoping they can eventually slide in the back door and be allowed to prescribe drugs.

CHAPTER 44

We Sat in the Same Classes—
We Heard the Same Thing

Earlier, we discussed that the purpose of licensing laws and state boards that regulate the rules is to protect the public. Therefore, when Dr. Jim insisted that we should be called chiropractic physicians or doctors of chiropractic medicine, this is very misleading and confusing. It does not accurately portray the unique service that chiropractors provide. Let's go back to our Rhode Island friend trying to send her friend in Chicago to a chiropractor who adjusts the spine. She wants her friend to receive a good adjustment. It should appear logical that chiropractors who graduate from the same school studying the same thing would adjust you when you went to them. Dr. Jim and I went to the same school, and you would assume we would be doing the same thing. When you go to a dentist, they do one thing. Medical doctors generally dispense the same drugs. But if you go to one of Dr. Jim's graduates, aligning your hips, leveling your sacrum, and straightening your spine will not be their primary goal, if addressed at all. They will give you a medical exam, a medical diagnosis, and then prescribe one of the many holistic or medical therapies that they think will parallel what they believe the medics would do.

This is not the practice of chiropractic; this is the practice of half-assed medicine mixed with chiropractic, or what Dr. Jim calls chiropractic medicine, and it is an entirely different animal. It does have chiropractic in its name, and that is what is misleading because when you see the word chiropractic, you associate it with an adjustment.

The policy of forcing chiropractors into chiropractic medicine with its diversification and even pushing for the right to prescribe drugs leads to incompetence. Providers doing a little of this and a little of that do not necessarily ensure quality care for the public. I am not sure how Dr. Jim and others in chiropractic today justify the drive for diversification. I know that Dr. Jim is knowledgeable. Maybe I was sleeping in class when he heard what he did about diversification. What I heard from the instructors was to be the best-darned adjustor you can be. Dr. Janse, our president, admonished us in every convocation we had to learn how to adjust the first cervical vertebrae to help headaches. He would say, "If you get good at adjusting it, you will have people lined up all the way to King Arthur's," which was a restaurant about two hundred yards from the school. I never once heard him say that we needed to push drugs.

I took Dr. Janse's advice and learned, as did Dr. Jim under Dr. Alfred States, our technique instructor, how to give a proper adjustment. That is what I have been doing for the last fifty years. There is no diversification in our office and never has been. The people know what they are going to get, and they come prepared to get their hips checked. They know what the fee will be and that there are no hidden costs. They know we have an open-door policy, and they have to sign in and wait for their turn. We are open seven days a week, and they know we have an honest place where you can come and go without any hassle.

We have a broad industrial base in the area, and the people who work in these factories want to get in and out and back to work as fast as possible. We make it easy for them; we give an exceptional adjustment as Dr. States taught us. When you provide a proper adjustment, great things happen. Most chiropractors struggle for new patients because of Dr. Jim's and other leaders of the profession's policies that make chiropractic into something other than what it is.

To be successful, you have to treat people like you would want to be treated and be honest. We have sustained a high number of new patients every week for fifty-two years. If we can keep that pace for all these years, there should be no reason the profession should be seeing only a small percentage of the population. What an irony, Dr. Jim learned from the same instructors that I did and he became one of the world's leaders in chiropractic, yet his policies allow the chiropractors to see 5 percent of the population. I go out the same door with the same diploma as he has, and the theories I learned under the same instructors allows me to see 30 percent of my community. It is both ironic and yet sad that more of the public doesn't have access to chiropractic.

CHAPTER 45

The Two Faces of Chiropractic

After fifty years of practicing and observing chiropractic, my assessment of why you cannot get a good chiropractic adjustment that would help you and your family with your health care is because of our educational system. This educational format is the biggest perpetrator of the problem. Doctoral schools were designed to make specialists experts in their field. Specialists do, in fact, zero in on their specialty. Therefore, if chiropractic schools bestow a doctoral degree on each of its graduates, how can Dr. Jim and I hear the same professors who taught the same things to both of us day in and day out yet come out of the same school with two different "faces"? How did Dr. Jim embrace Dr. Howard's theory that chiropractic should be another item in the doctor's black bag, and I heard the call that we should spend our time adjusting the whole world?

This phenomenon is what is happening in every chiropractic college in America, not just at National College. Every chiropractic school has an educational system that is creating and developing two personalities for their graduates. The profession has a split personality; it does not know what it is and hasn't known for the last 120 years. It mixes medicine and chiropractic and comes out with a chiropractic physician or a doctor of chiropractic medicine, which are oxymorons, a complete contradiction in terms.

The doctorate of the chiropractic profession makes a mockery of the universally accepted doctoral degree. If you would poll the chiropractors, most of them on either side of the fence would agree that it is tough to explain to the public the various forms of chiropractic. If my classmate, Dr. Jim, and I were put in front of a panel and ask to discuss chiropractic education to prospective students, prospective patients, people from the insurance, or governmental agencies, what would be our explanation? How would we describe how we studied the same material and received an identical diploma, but the doctorate Dr. Jim received expanded and diversified his direction and the one I received narrowed mine? I would suspect our audience would walk away from our discussion baffled and shaking their heads.

For over a hundred years, my profession could have been helping all of humanity. Instead, you have had to suffer because of this division.

Doctoral education is designed to continually narrow the focus of the students, which automatically allows for quality outcomes and defines their expertise. Chiropractic's doctoral education flies in the face of the universal doctoral programs and does the opposite. Chiropractic expands instead of narrowing, and it is not working. It has not worked and will not work in the future if the format remains the same. It allows us to see so few of the population when we have the knowledge and talent to see the majority. When this scenario exists, there is a problem, and common sense would say this problem needs to be rectified.

People may scoff at the squatty potty, but for some it really works!

SQUATTY POTTY

Try losing some weight by placing your feet on a box when you defecate.

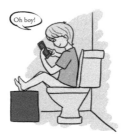 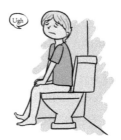

Our large intestine has a right angle at its base.

When we sit on the stool with our feet on the floor, we eliminate roughly 8 inches.

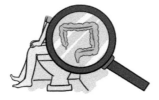 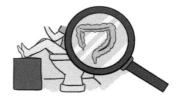

When we elevate our legs and feet, we straighten the right angle and eliminate up to 16 inches.

Enough said!

CHAPTER 46

Education—Using Lou Holtz's Philosophy

Chiropractic needs to join this century in how it educates our doctors. My experience of receiving a bachelor's degree from a college that specialized in education, along with teaching in the public school system for two years, has given me a different insight than most. In addition to my fifty years of practice experience, I sat on a chiropractic college board for twelve years, chairing it for ten years. It is my conclusion that chiropractic's greatest obstacle and the primary reason chiropractors are taking care of so few of you is that the curriculum format is *wrong*!

The format is upside down from mainline/universal educational programs. Many chiropractors have never had any mainline comprehensive educational experience. Initially, chiropractors were only required to have a high school education to enter school. Today, many schools only require a two-year college prerequisite, and those two years are primarily required science courses. The chiropractic schools have traditionally modeled chiropractic coursework after medical schools and the preparation for the national and state chiropractic board examinations. Chiropractic schools then proceed to teach the students every modality and technique under the sun. I will guarantee that any curriculum director or expert from any one of our state colleges or universities will agree that there needs to be a wholesale change.

Chiropractic is the only profession that does not adhere to the accepted standard of three segmental steps in the doctoral candidate requirement procedure. In every doctoral program, you have to prove yourself before you can move on to the next level. The first step all pro-grams require is a bachelor's degree with a certain grade-point level plus good standing with the law and other statutes. The chiropractic profes-sion rarely requires a bachelor's degree, nor do they require background checks. Most chiropractic schools require only two years of prerequisite courses with a minimum passing grade.

The main reason the mainline universal doctoral programs orig-inated was to produce experts. What is the purpose of becoming an expert? An expert narrows the field and learns all necessary facts and minutiae about the subject matter. By pinpointing a subject and learn-ing all relevant material assure that no stone has been left unturned. The designers of the doctoral program wanted this narrowing to ensure qual-ity control. Quality control was a prominent issue when the designers of the educational programs were set up by the Carnegie Educational Foundation in the 1920s and '30s.

Chiropractors skip the first segment in this normal progression for the doctorate that mainline schools require. Chiropractic schools only need two years of college to enter their program. Mainline schools require a bachelor's with at least a B average to enable the candidate to move into the master's degree program, which is the second segment in the standard degree progression. Chiropractors do not have a master's program and allow their candidates to go directly into their five-year or ten-semester doctoral syllabus with only a two-year prerequisite.

Most educational counselors will tell you that the bachelor's pro-gram is not entirely about the degree that you receive but that you have stayed the course and finished the prescribed program satisfactorily and successfully. Statistics show that nine out of ten graduates change fields somewhere along the line, many exiting the area in which they majored. Most counselors will say that the four-year program is more of a growth and maturation period. It is a period away from the pressure of parents and before the scrutiny of a spouse. It is a time when decisions are made on your own. Lou Holtz, the famous football coach, tells how first-year students come in scared, sophomores work hard, juniors have fun, and seniors are ready to meet the challenge that awaits and for, which they have been preparing. College is a time of carefree responsibility. You need to work on your studies, have some fun, participate in new and different activities without parents or siblings looking over your shoulder. It is a time of learning how to discipline yourself and others around you. It is a time to get *it* out of your system.

It is a time to study liberal arts and listen to far-out professors tell you things you never heard at home. It is a time to discuss these ideas and decide what is practical or impractical. It is a time to live in a dormitory with hundreds of others, share living space, bathrooms, and eating facilities away from parents and family. It is a time to join fraternities and sororities where you learn social skills, leadership, and perform community service to give and help others.

Four years of college is the only time you are really by yourself. Before college, it was your mother, father, or siblings who were always around. After college, it will be a husband or a wife being present. It is a growth period that everyone should experience. At the end of four years, you have a degree. You are ready for work, you have grown through four years of maturation, and you have climbed the mountain. You did it. You made the decisions, and you accomplished it all on your own!

CHAPTER 47

Missed Experience

The chiropractic profession unfortunately does not allow or require their candidates the luxury of four years of maturation. Chiropractic education fails their candidates by depriving them of this space of time to develop and mature socially. Social maturation is vitally important to any specialist because, as a specialist, you become an authority, and authorities need to understand how to work with people. Chiropractic students attend a school that requires sitting in class thirty hours per week to complete the mandated course of study. There is no time for them to mature socially.

Unfortunately, these maturation years are not a part of the pre-requisite chiropractic curriculum. Chiropractic students who want to be ALA chiropractors—those who align, level, and adjust—will choose the two-year path because they want to get out and get into practice. They are not interested in being pseudomedics. Unfortunately, they become prey to becoming pseudomedics because they do not have enough maturity, social experience, or life's knowledge to say no to the wannabes that run the profession. (How can they say no? They are in school and have to do as taught to graduate.) The wannabes say you must become a chiropractic physician to be accepted in your commu-nity. Students come into chiropractic with high hopes of being a darned good chiropractor but are insecure and feel inadequate without other options. If they had gotten a bachelor's degree in business or biology, it would give them confidence if they didn't make it as a straight chiropractor. It is regrettable for anyone to have to change from what they had their heart set on, adjusting patients, to becoming something else because of the missed opportunity of social growth.

CHAPTER 48

Wannabes Being Unfair

Most wannabe medics who get involved in chiropractic schools will usually come in with a bachelor's degree. Ninety-five percent of the wannabees had their heart set on being a medical doctor but could not get into medical school. They will tell you that they were accepted, but for some reason, they decided not to go. They have a bachelor's degree when they enter chiropractic school because it is a medical school requirement.

These medical school washouts make it difficult for a two-year student that wants to be a chiropractor. These wannabes become the bullies. The wannabees come into chiropractic to be a "real doctor," and they want to change chiropractic into chiropractic medicine and dispense drugs. They want to make chiropractic scientifically acceptable. They like the idea of Dr. Jim's doctor of chiropractic medicine. They never wanted to adjust; they want to be like "real" doctors and are trying very hard to make chiropractic into the medical image of what they think it should be. They have little tolerance for the straight chiropractor. The vast majority of two-year people will be intimidated and harassed into becoming a mixer. You enter chiropractic school believing you can become a chiropractor, but you are converted and become a half-assed medic, a chiropractic physician.

It is unfair to the student that wanted to be a chiropractor who aligns hips, levels sacrums, and adjusts the spine. But it is also unjust to the public. You will not have a chiropractor to adjust you, your friends, and your community. This young chiropractor will be a chiropractic physician performing acupuncture, physical therapy, laser, nutritional and weight reduction counseling, smoking cessation, and oriental medicine.

CHAPTER 49

BJ's Role in the Educational Format

When BJ started his first school in 1904, all he wanted was a warm body and enough money for six months of tuition. BJ would say he could make a good chiropractor a damn good chiropractor in six months. He did not want additional education. That was okay for the first twenty years. However, when the medics started forcing more college on the profession, BJ did not go along with the times. He thought more education would lead to more medical education, and of course, he was correct. BJ was a great visionary, but he missed the boat on how to protect and set up his doctoral program.

An ALA straight chiropractor is possibly one of the most important ways to help keep a person healthy that exists today. It is a vitally important way to stay well. If the profession has this responsibility, it needs a conventional doctoral program to allow the public to get the most exceptional, most qualified care they can obtain.

A student needs to learn where, when, and how to adjust. They need to know the body inside and out and be able to visualize the spine and hips and how each facet joint works and operates. They also need to be aware of the status of the patient's health and their history before an adjustment is given. Chiropractors need to learn the art of adjusting that is on par with becoming a concert pianist. To become a primary ALA chiropractor, I believe students need three years of concentrated study. BJ said six months was sufficient, and he did not want more education. Even though he was the authority, I disagree on the basis that we need a bachelor's degree for maturation and social graces as well as having a backup field in case chiropractic does not pan out for someone or an injury occurs. We do not need more medical education; we need three years of concentrated chiropractic study. A student who has received a bachelor's degree will be able to accept the ALA curriculum and become a great adjuster. If it turns out adjusting is not their cup of tea, they have a degree they can fall back on.

BJ discussed the idea of change. Without change, things stagnate and deteriorate. Chiropractic has had more medical education forced on them, which is precisely what BJ was afraid would happen. Change is necessary to correct BJ's mistakes and to throw out much of the unnecessary medical education that was forced upon us that does not pertain to chiropractic. It is time to stop being hostages to the medics and be taught to become the very best chiropractors we can be from a chiropractic standpoint.

CHAPTER 50

Common Sense Education

Earlier, we discussed that the medical, insurance, and government entities want chiropractic to be scientifically proven to become a legitimate player in health care and be able to justify paying their claims. We also discussed that chiropractic would never be shown to be scientific because you cannot experiment on a live, upright human being. Hitler tried it, and how did that turn out? Chiropractic deals with gravity and how the erect stance affects structural alignment.

There is a story that Einstein could not prove what gravity did to the human body. One day he was in front of a sizable audience discussing his scientific theories when he brought up the subject of gravity on the human body. He said he'd had this idea in mind for a long time because gravity's effect on the human body has never been measured and no experiments had ever been performed on an upright human body. He said, "Now just imagine an elevator full of people up thirty stories. We would cut the cables, letting the elevator free fall for those thirty stories and having a way to measure the effects of the gravity on their bodies as the people fell, when they stopped, and whatever whip back there would be." The crowd was shocked that he would suggest such an experiment, even if it were only in his thoughts.

This type of experiment is what is necessary if we are ever going to prove chiropractic. Still, it will never happen because we cannot do trial-and-error tests on upright human specimens in this manner. Even the great Einstein could not show what the effects of gravity did to the human spine. Therefore, without scientists being able to experiment on any of us while we are alive and upright, I feel that chiropractic will never be proven in the laboratory to be an absolute fact. Even though it cannot be established in the laboratory doesn't mean that it doesn't work. In my fifty-two years of practice, I have seen thousands upon thousands of patients respond favorably and effectively.

CHAPTER 51

Cohorts

Dr. Janse, National Chiropractic School's president, loved to quote the poet Rudyard Kipling, especially from "The Stranger." The last stanza begins, "This was my father's belief and this is also mine!" BJ was not concerned about scientific proof from a medical standpoint. He used to say if the ole cow cuts herself on a barbed wire fence and the cut is not too great to lose all her pressure, the wound will heal. What scientific proof is necessary to understand this concept? The same is true with the vertebral subluxation. If the vertebra is not too far out of place to cause breakage or herniation, the subluxation can be corrected, and healing will take place. I agree with BJ, and to paraphrase Kipling, he was a man of my own stock. Bitter bad he may be, but at least, he heard the things I heard and saw the things I saw. BJ Palmer believed it, and so do I!

BJ Palmer would say that when a subluxation exists, it blocks the life force from the brain to the tissue cell. The result of this blockage causes the tissue or cell not to function as it was intended. The subluxation is corrected when the bone is manually adjusted into motion sending it from point B back to its original point A. With this correction, the blockage is removed and the life force will again be able to flow freely. This life force, as it flows freely, allows the innate forces, the unseen forces that run throughout bodies, to take over and restore health to the body.

BJ Palmer developed the chiropractic philosophy based on this subluxation, the adjustment of the subluxation, and the innate intelligence that is associated with restoring the life force that flows over the nerves. BJ wrote thirty-nine books, the majority based on this idea, which is a simple, unique, and common-sense concept demonstrating the importance structure plays in health. If we do not possess a reasonable semblance of excellent structure, we will have deteriorating health and longevity problems.

Most of BJ's books are buried in the archives because they are politically incorrect and are embarrassing to the elites of the mixing wannabe ranks. BJ is a closet case to the elites.

The irony is that the elite wannabes want to be sophisticated and scientific, but they all have massage therapy signs in their practices. Massage parlors and science do not travel in the same circles. My friend, Dr. Jim, the advocate of chiropractic/medicine, was the first to bring a massage school into his program. This group of chiropractors was distraught with BJ and his association with the innate intelligence factor or what they call pseudo-religious jargon. In essence, the mixing element of chiropractic treats the philosophic or straight chiropractors as country cousins. Remember the cousin you could not stand but would come to stay a week during the summer with your mother's invitation? When your friends came, you did not want to be associated with your cousin because they were an embarrassment, they did not fit in, and you would have loved to have been able to stick them in a closet until your guests were gone. The wannabes are ashamed of their country cousin BJ and his theory that once the interference to a nerve has been removed by adjusting a subluxated vertebra, then the innate intelligence of the body will take over and alleviate the dis-ease. Yet it is okay to have massage therapists in their offices!

CHAPTER 52

BJ's Mythical Sky Jockey

The mixers do not agree with Palmer's brand of chiropractic. They say it is unscientific and borders on religion. When Palmer talked of innate intelligence as the power that made us and is also the power that heals us, the wannabees get out of sorts because of his quasireligious philosophy, which they feel only the ignorant would believe. The wannabees believe science is what heals, and the drugs manufactured by the pharmaceutical companies are what heals, not the innate intelligence of the body. They think Palmer's philosophy and concept of chiropractic is pure hogwash.

Ironically, the mixer wannabees, with all their complaining about Palmer, have never written a book of guidelines that spell out what chiropractic is or is not. All they tend to write about is how unfair it is that they cannot diversify and broaden the scope of chiropractic to include prescribing medication.

BJ's Green Books are the foundation of chiropractic. He wrote extensively, and it is a crying shame that his books are not readily available and that the world does not have access to and an opportunity to read them. Without BJ's books as a guide, there is nothing written on chiropractic that gives the profession a solid direction as to what the profession stands for or the direction it should be heading. In other words, the elites have buried chiropractic's constitution. What would travel be like if we took the white line from the middle of the road? Mass chaos would ensue with everyone going their way, causing slow travel time and a very unproductive system of travel.

The wannabees have gained control of our schools and are destroying the foundation of chiropractic by removing its white line, which allows for more diversity, more therapies, and more chaos. They are supposed to be intelligent leaders, but they have no ideas of their own other than to plagiarize and mimic the medics. This thinking and policy is broadening the practice of chiropractic to the point that it does not have any boundaries. "Good fences make good neighbors" is an old saying that holds true. Chiropractic has no fences, no boundaries, and as a result, no discipline. Unfortunately, those who suffer from this liberal thinking is yes, you, the public. Chiropractors spend more time trying to figure out how to extort $3,000 or $4,000 out of your insurance policy than they will on how to best adjust you. Sadly, it is all about them and not you.

Action on the part of chiropractic educational institutions to broaden the doctoral process is not what the mainline and universal educators have in mind for postgraduate degrees. Specialists have strict fences and have to follow narrow channels, or they could never become a specialist.

BJ wanted the profession to be specialists with fences, but medical school washouts hijacked his program. He wanted his students to understand the Palmer chiropractic philosophy thoroughly. A philosophy based on a quasireligious component. Chiropractors adjust a misaligned vertebra releasing it to reset into its proper function and alignment, allowing the energy force to flow again as God designed so normalcy can return.

Palmer's philosophy is still taught in some of our chiropractic schools but not in the mixing schools. Even in the schools that have it in their curriculum, it is watered down. In hindsight, it may have been better if BJ had used a term other than philosophy. He wanted it to be a doctrine but instead designated it a philosophy. Philosophies, as taught in liberal arts schools, are not taught as doctrine. They are not laid out as a direction to live by; their presentation is food for thought.

Palmer wanted his philosophy to be a way of life, and philosophies cannot work this way. For example, Spinosa and some of the other greats who are studied in liberal art classrooms are meant to be discussed, digested, spit out, and wallowed around in until finally, something practical may be gleaned from their ideas. Still, most often, they are introduced to shake up a student's thinking.

CHAPTER 53

Four versus Two

Herein lies a problem with the chiropractic two-year prerequisite requirement; the student comes to school with no liberal arts philosophy under their belt. When they are introduced to the Palmer philosophy, they wind up treating it like it was a liberal arts philosophy course. They want to chew on it, tear it apart, examine it, and make mincemeat out of Palmer's thinking. They scrutinize it, trying to find loopholes in it when they should be at the point of accepting it and using it for their bedrock because they already had a liberal arts philosophy background. Instead, they start to question their foundation. It is when they start questioning and no longer agree with Palmer's theories that they drift into a mindset that exists in chiropractic regarding innate intelligence. Real doctors do not believe like this; therefore, it is foolish. It is at this point, if they are not grounded in common sense and do not have a bachelor's degree to fall back on, they begin listening to the wannabes in their class and change their goal of being a chiropractor to that of a chiropractic physician.

Once the two-year liberal arts student gives up their principle, they begin sliding toward the mixer's thinking. Chances are, they will graduate and go out and practice like the wannabe medics because they are now convinced that they would be more acceptable to the public.

If they had a four-year degree, they would possibly not have caved into the wannabes, because of the security of their bachelor's degree to fall back on if necessary. However, coming into chiropractic school with only two years of prerequisites, there is no safety net. As they continue with five years of chiropractic school, they will graduate having only one degree in seven years of education and only one venue. Since this degree is only useful in chiropractic, not many businesses will want to hire you with only a chiropractic degree. Therefore, if you find you do not like the practice of chiropractic or you try and fail, you have nothing to fall back on. What a grave predicament for the profession. It is terrible for our schools to have allowed this to happen.

Recently a young graduate came to visit my office. He told me he had been out of school for five years and that nothing was working for him. Because of this, he had given up on chiropractic and had applied to the post office for a job. Later, I heard that he is now carrying mail for a local post office. He had no backup degree, no safety net, yet he had a six-year degree that has no value in the business world. Six long years and $200,000 incurred in student loans for tuition down the drain. Could this be called white-collar crime committed by our schools? It should be! If we have a 50 percent failure rate in chiropractic after five years in practice, something is problematic in our educational system! We are not doing justice to our graduates under the current educational format.

The young fellow I mentioned told me that every chiropractic physician he worked for insisted that he hard sell patients a twenty-five- to thirty-visit package, with three or four therapies included, and wanted him to get the patient to pay in advance for these services. That is the Parker practice building procedure that we have previously discussed and has been used by the profession for the past sixty years. It takes an excellent salesperson to work this scheme. If you do not have a sophisticated sales ability, then the practice of chiropractic is not going to be exciting or profitable. He wanted to be a chiropractor and adjust the spine; he did not want to be a salesman and could not sell things to people that he thought they did not need. He was fed up with the sales aspect of chiropractic. I told him that he could observe me and watch how we take care of patients. We never have to sell anyone anything. You never have to sell or coerce patients when you give them an exceptional adjustment at a fee the working people can afford. It is fun, and people love it. If you treat people the way you would want to be treated, everyone wins. Any chiropractor, who uses this patient-care method and puts the patient first will have people beating a path to their door and knocking the door down to receive this service. Under these circumstances, you are adjusting patients who are excited that they have a place to come for relief and support, making it fun to go to the office every day.

Our unsuccessful young chiropractor did come to watch me for a couple of days but said, "Nah, I'm too burned out. I am going to pursue a job at the Post Office." How sad. It made me angry at our educational system for spending his time, taking his tuition money, and putting him out on the street without a success plan, thereby letting him fail. These young graduates should not have to fail, but if they do, it not only hurts them but all of you. If the school had taught him how to manage patients properly, he would be in the field today (along with all our other failing graduates). They all could be seeing hundreds of patients, keeping all of you from suffering needlessly, and making this world a better place to live. Our chiropractic educational institutions should feel guilty and ashamed.

CHAPTER 54

Growth Period

In reality, all chiropractic students should have a growth period of four years spent studying a liberal arts curriculum. Chiropractic schools should not accept anyone who has not had the life experience of a bachelor's degree. It could be a degree in any field. If after they have been in school and decide it is not for them or if they are in the field become injured or it does not work out for them, they have been trained in another area and have something to fall back on.

The four-year diploma shows a person's perseverance and patience. It shows that they made a decision, stuck with it, and finished the course, demonstrating character and strength. More importantly, it gave them time to mature. Maturity, along with common sense, is what we like to see exhibited in a potential chiropractic student. We are not looking for brilliance; we want hardworking students who can accept the chiropractic philosophy and not want to change the philosophy. We want compassionate students with empathy for others, who are not obsessed with money and understand that we should be helping all of humanity. We want thousands of students who are excited about giving beneficial adjustments at an affordable fee and who will treat their patients as they would want to be treated.

With few exceptions, we all begin, as the old Ivory Snow commercial stated, "99 and 44/100 percent pure." Medicine and science alter the body using substances from outside the body. Because those outside factors force changes in the body that can be measured, that change becomes defined as science. Chiropractic deals with a body that has been altered by an external force, usually in the form of trauma or a repetitive work action. The chiropractor levers the misaligned vertebrae or hip back to its normal position and then leaves it to God's power to heal through the body's innate intelligence, to take over and allow the healing to occur. Chiropractic and medicine are opposites. Medicine alters the body using outside forces, attempting to return the body to normal. Chiropractic adjusts the structure, setting vertebra in motion to allow the body to return to normal. This premise needs to be accepted in full faith by chiropractors.

Questioning philosophical tenets should have been completed in undergraduate school. Once the degreed bachelor student arrives at chiropractic school, they will have grown, matured, and sown their wild oats, believing that chiropractic would be a good fit and a bright future for them. Should circumstances change for them, they will still be marketable with the bachelor's degree they earned in undergraduate school.

CHAPTER 55

The Educational Reformation—
Stop Nero from Fiddling

Educational reform is a critical issue. It is what hampered my profession for over one hundred years. The past and present educational format does not work as it should. Our forefathers, Washington and Jefferson, et. al., were adamant that if we do not educate the common man, it will not be long before the strong overtake the weak as happened in Europe. In the early 1900s, Carnegie and the government overhauled the educational system from top to bottom, and it has worked quite well until recently. Our forefathers would be appalled by the way we are toying with two or more languages in our country. They were firm about wanting only one language. They argued that if we have two or three languages, we will begin fighting as they did in Europe two hundred years ago and are still doing today because of the language barrier. When people do not understand one another, it is frustrating and can lead to many problems, including war.

A language problem exists in chiropractic, and it is a serious one. It is the main reason all of you are not being taken care of by chiropractors as should be happening. Unfortunately, all chiropractors seem to do is fight. One side talks one language, and the other side talks another resulting in discord. One group declares that to be a chiropractor, you have to do it this way, and they work to have a law passed stating it has to be done this way. The other group lobbies to do it their way and accuses the other side of undermining them.

In the last ten years, we now have a group calling themselves doctors of chiropractic medicine. They, along with the chiropractic physicians and the straight chiropractors, all came out of the same school. How can this be? What does the school's curriculum consist of that doctors come out headed in three different directions, using different languages? I want to challenge any mainline curriculum expert to examine the chiropractic syllabus to see how this can occur. One school with three separate designations for the same degree is very confusing. The profession is akin to Europe with its many languages.

More advancements and improvements in humankind's standard of living have come from America, where we speak one language and understand what one another is saying. Everything works smoother when we can communicate, share, and not have to interpret. Sharing a common language gives us the ability to help one another expand, progress, and become successful.

It would be great if our profession spoke one language that would unite us. Dentists use the same vocabulary, as do medics, osteopaths, and podiatrists. Straight chiropractic utilized the subluxation and the adjustment of that subluxation as its basis. Think of straight chiropractic as a ship that is sailing the mighty ocean. It carries the payload but over time has accumulated barnacles and each barnacle flies its flag. There is an acupuncture flag, a banner for physical therapy, one for nutritionists, a flag for oriental medicine, a big one for laser therapy, and flags for other therapies. If we aren't diligent soon, there could be one flying for drug therapy. That old ship loaded with barnacles will continue to slow the growth rate for chiropractic.

CHAPTER 56

The Solution for Diversification

To solve the diversification problem that exists in chiropractic today, let's use a solution that has been around for a long time and used by all other professions. If we want to become like the medics, then we better copy their doctoral plan and use it for our students. Therefore, the chiropractic doctorate program would consist of the following:

1.) The requirement of a bachelor's degree in any field to enter chiropractic college. Prerequisites of one basic physics course and two philosophy courses. An entrance question involving the student's life experience and how it would blend with the purpose and philosophy of chiropractic.
2.) Three academic years of preparation for a general doctor of chiropractic degree. Courses in preparatory knowledge of normal and abnormal body function to include
   A. Anatomy
   B. Physiology
   C. Pathology
   D. Physics, human structure

Courses in applied knowledge include

   A. Chiropractic philosophy as related to structural physics
   B. Body analysis as related to structural physics

C. Vertebral adjusting technique as related to structure of the body

3.) National or State Board Examinations would be administered to test the candidate's understanding of the above material.

4.) Chiropractic candidates must complete the above course requirements and pass the board material to become a competent full spine chiropractor.

5.) Once the first three-year commitment is satisfied the graduate may do the following:

A. enter the field and practice as a doctor of Chiropractic that adjusts the joints of the body.

B. For those who wish to use specialized techniques of adjusting, such as activator, instrument adjusting, or other therapies such as physical therapy, acupuncture, script writing, oriental medicine, laser therapy, weight loss, and nutritional wellness programs, they would be required to attend two more years of study beyond the three-year basic course of chiropractic.

6.) By completing a two-year on-campus residency and studying these therapy courses in a legitimate academic setting will give credibility to the chiropractic physician degree. (Today many of these courses are taught on weekends in hotel conference rooms.)

7.) Upon completion of these two years of specialty study, the title of chiropractic physician would be bestowed on the candidate once board examinations covering these therapies have been passed successfully.

What Would This Solve?

1. This doctoral format would emulate other professions, giving chiropractors an equal degree.

2. By identifying what the chiropractor has specialized in will eliminate misunderstanding of what the patient will be receiving.
3. Identify the straight chiropractor and the chiropractic physician as separate and distinct.

Some chiropractors who read this will say, "Wait, the chiropractic physicians will know how to adjust as I do, and they will think they are better than me." Once all chiropractors are required to have a bachelor's degree before their doctorate, if they are not satisfied with adjusting only and want to perform therapies, they can return to campus for two additional years of residency and become a chiropractic physician. The chiropractic doctoral program needs revamping so that there are fences and boundaries and the public will know what they will be receiving.

Just as the chiropractic curriculum needs to be changed, our bodies need to be flushed out on a regular basis.

MORNING WATER

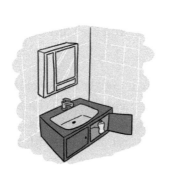
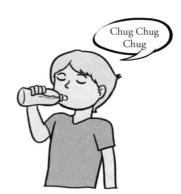

Keep a 20 oz bottle of water on your bathroom sink cabinet.

Chug it down immediately. Forcing 20 oz rids the body of debris that accumulated over night. It purges the system like using the water hose to flush your cars radiator.

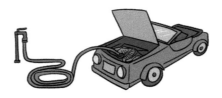

Once you have washed your self out, now have your coffee.

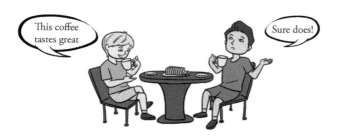
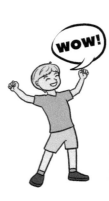

Try it, elevating your water level right away will make you feel better all day.

CHAPTER 57

The End Result of Reorganization

Most candidates coming to chiropractic school with a bachelor's degree will accept that it is the subluxation of the vertebrae and the adjustment of that subluxation, which allows chiropractic to exist and be licensed. The first three years of chiropractic school will concentrate on understanding the normal function of the body as well as abnormal function. Second, they will learn the physics of the mechanical part of the body, how it works, how it can be misaligned, and how it can be corrected. Thirdly, a thorough understanding of the adjusting techniques that will be utilized in the correction of misalignments and subluxations will be taught and practiced so that the student becomes a master at adjusting.

I have used the straight chiropractic adjustment procedure for over fifty years and still look forward to going to the office every day to see patients. Some patients will need to be referred to another practitioner. Approximately 80 percent will respond favorably to the initial adjustment. Still, 20 percent will require additional work, and some of this group may have let the problem go too long to receive results. If there were a chiropractic physician in my area, trained in the manner I have suggested, I would refer any nonresponding patient to them. How wonderful it would be to have someone who could help patients conservatively and alternatively and not merely write a prescription for drugs. This is my vision for the future.

If two thirds of chiropractors were aligning hips, leveling sacrums, and adjusting the spine at an affordable fee, this atmosphere would create a venue that would allow chiropractors to start seeing over 50 percent of the population. These chiropractors could refer patients who need additional care to chiropractic physicians who would utilize therapeutic knowledge along with their adjusting skills to care for them. This would be a win-win situation for the patient, the straight chiropractor, and the chiropractic physician.

Another area that chiropractic physicians could capitalize on is a by-product of the medical profession. Medical doctors and drug companies are market makers. Earlier I used the example of the school teacher who was retiring and went in for an exam, thinking it was a good idea to begin his retirement in the best possible shape. The medics testing found his prostate could prove to be a problem and decided to take care of it immediately. They took care of it, and he now has chronic low back pain and has to wear a diaper. The medical profession is producing one chronic problem after another. This would not have had to happen. When stockholders want returns on their investments, someone has to consume those drugs. All of you can name someone who has wound up with a medically induced problem. Each year, thousands and thousands are added to the role of chronic-pain patients, those who desperately need access to nonpharmacological health care services. It is hard to believe that the amount of oxycontin prescribed for severe chronic pain is enough for every man, woman, and child in the United States to have a daily supply for one and one half months!

In talking with your friends and relatives, have you noticed how many have had major surgery and then been hung out to dry. Once the heart, cancer, back, or knee surgeries are done, according to the surgeons, they have "fixed" your problem. You are cured. I have noticed in my practice, back or knee operations are helpful for the first two years, then the old problem begins creeping back in. Recurring pain now becomes the tale of woe I hear from patients. The operating surgeon will not discuss it with you. Remember they fixed it. They send you back to your general practitioner. The GP sends you back to physical therapy, which you completed shortly after the operation. This proves to be unsatisfactory. The patient will be hustled to pain management. Once you get to pain management, I think you know that it is at this point—they have pretty well given up on you! This then is where the oxycontin prescriptions come into play. You are now labeled a chronic-pain patient. There are millions of chronic-pain patients who need help, but they need more help than being addicted to oxycontin.

The chiropractic physicians need to tap into this market that the medics have created. The medics are not taking care of it and are clueless, other than giving more drugs. All these medical failures could be acres of diamonds in the chiropractic physician's backyard.

What a future the profession could have by restructuring the chiropractic curriculum and focusing on areas where there is the greatest need. Chiropractors could be adjusting the working masses, while the chiropractic physicians could become the caretakers, specialists, and authorities for the patients the doctor of chiropractic could not handle. With their adjustive skills and numerous medical therapies, the chiropractic physicians could take over the medical failure patients, giving them an alternative to prescription drugs. Why should we accept being called quacks when we could become saints by merely restructuring our educational format?

CHAPTER 58

The Gender Gap

There is another situation that has evolved in the past number of years that needs to be addressed. It deals with women in chiropractic. In the last couple of decades, the female enrollment in our chiropractic schools has increased to a fifty-fifty ratio. This ratio is changing the landscape of our chiropractic practice to include more and more therapies. The reason for adding more therapies is due to the lack of physical strength of women.

The original Diversified full spine adjusting technique that made chiropractic popular with the eighteen- to sixty-five-year-old work-ing people is because they like to feel the vertebrae moving while an adjustment is taking place. This technique will get 80 percent of the working people back on the job in no time. However, it is heavy-duty work, not a lot different than working in a factory setting. Adjusting is manual labor and is one of the reasons the profession uses adjusting guns and computer techniques to get away from manual adjusting. This can become a problem with a 110-pound female trying to adjust a 220-pound worker. Diversified adjusting is vigorous and takes a lot of brawn to expedite. Very few smaller women have the physical strength or height for leverage to properly perform these adjustments.

Chiropractic is heavy work. There is finesse in an adjustment. It is a combination of pushing, pulling, thrusting, levering and prying in one deft move. I liken it to taking an apple off a tree. You can reach up to grab the apple and pull the apple and limb toward you, which by force will tear off the apple. Or you can take the apple, turn it until the tension is tight, then with a quick, deft inferior pull, snap it free. The deft part is not difficult for women, but taking to tension a 220-pound person to the point of using the critical deft maneuver to move the vertebrae is where the 110-pound women may find difficulty. As the old-timers would say, she is "too light in the seat."

An example of being "too light" happened recently. We have a female chiropractor in our area that tries her best to compete with the brawny men. A patient, Jim, went to see her three months ago complaining of right hip pain. He is thirty-six years old, 180 pounds, and does heavy, difficult work in our local trailer-RV industry. A local chiropractor we will call Dr. Sandy accepted him as a patient and tried to move his hip using the Diversified approach. According to Jim, she was "too light in the seat" to get his hip to adjust. Since that did not work, she used an adjusting gun that hammers like a small jackhammer. Dr. Sandy explained to Jim that this approach should break the stuck joint loose allowing it to slide back into place. She also used laser therapy, physical therapy, and gave him a massage.

Each of the four days he went to her that week, he received the same routine. Over the weekend, there was no improvement in his condition. He decided to go to his medic, who gave him pain pills and muscle relaxers. After a few days of taking those medications, he still had no improvement.

A buddy stopped by to see how he was getting along, found he wasn't doing well, and encouraged him to come to our office. Jim checked in on a Monday, and we discovered his hip high on the right. Further examination indicated a healthy-looking specimen with no notable red flags, so we proceeded in leveling his hips. We adjusted him with the Diversified technique, which allows the patient to feel and hear the bone go into place. It is a tough adjustment to administer because it takes a substantial push to take the tension out of the joint, a strong thrust to open the joint, then a deft turn of the joint in the correct direction. All these have to be done simultaneously.

After a rest period, we checked his hips in the mirror, and both hips were now level. This leveling impressed Jim. After walking around the office for three or four minutes, he could not believe that 80 percent of the pressure was gone.

His medic had slated him off work for the third week. On Tuesday, he laid around the house all day. Wednesday, he came to our office all smiles because he was pain-free. Jim's situation is only one of the many cases across the country (and world) that demonstrates the importance of structure to health and well-being to working people as well as the general population. Just because we cannot see structural misalignment is no reason to give a drug stressing that this pill will make you feel better in a couple of days or setting patients up with a plethora of different therapies.

Jim was extremely pleased to be free of the physical pain, but he was not happy with the bill that he received from Dr. Sandy. She charged him $265 per visit for four visits, totaling $1,060. He said, "This makes me feel ill again. I will have to pay this out of my pocket, and it did not do me one bit of good."

This situation was not good for the profession, the patient, or Dr. Sandy. It was not good for her reputation; it was not beneficial for positive feedback or referrals. She received no satisfaction from trying to help him; it was a failure for her and the patient.

I feel sorry for Dr. Sandy, but I blame the chiropractic schools for putting her and her female colleagues in the position of having to compete in the field with stronger men. The schools have no shame of taking $200,000 in tuition money from women and not providing a niche for them to practice in and then making them compete physically with men.

It is high time for the profession to change this discrimination and injustice against women in chiropractic. The change that is necessary and could provide a niche for the women is the 4-3-2 curriculum alternative we have been discussing. In this scenario, women would have a place where their unique talents in health care could be utilized to their full capacity.

To reiterate,

1. Before entering chiropractic school, a bachelor's degree is required. What would happen if a chiropractor would become disabled or decide chiropractic is not for them? A bachelor's degree would give them something to fall back on.

2. The first three years of chiropractic school consists of learning the normal and the abnormal functions of the body and how to identify each. Finding and correcting subluxations using only Diversified standard core manual adjusting techniques. All other corrective methods and therapies are classified as specialties and will be taught in the second tier of the chiropractic curriculum. By concentrating only on the adjustment during the first three years, all chiropractic students will become extremely competent adjusters. At the end of these three years, those who wish to adjust only may leave and practice as a straight chiropractor, performing adjustments only.

3. The second phase to become a chiropractic physician will consist of two additional years on-campus learning specialty adjusting techniques and all therapies that are allowed under the present chiropractic licensing umbrella.

It is my opinion from fifty years of chiropractic practice that women need a niche. By encouraging them to go into the second tier and become authorities of our specialty techniques and therapies, they can specialize in helping the aged, the young, the chronic, and special needs patients. Women in chiropractic could excel in this area. Dr. Sandy could have used therapies on those who came to her that needed those specialties. She would not have had to accept Jim as a patient and try to handle something out of her physical realm.

Today no one knows what they are going to experience when they go to a chiropractor with all the different techniques, therapies and nutritional counseling that chiropractors offer. The 4-3-2 program can change this. It would be beneficial for Dr. Sandy, her patient Jim, the profession, and all potential patients to know which chiropractor to utilize. Patients need to know which chiropractor to go to for care to get back to work and who to see for more specialized needs.

The Future of Chiropractic versus the Future of Chiropractic

The Bible, in Proverbs 29:18, states, "Where there is no vision the people perish." Our leaders' vision is that of the hostage syndrome. When you read the chiropractic expert's version, there will not be a lot of hope for exceptional, affordable adjustments in their vision for the future.

Daniel Sosnoski, editor-in-chief of one of the largest chiropractic magazines, in an article titled "The Future Chiropractor" in the May 4, 2018, issue of *Chiropractic Economics* stated that all chiropractic experts agree that collaboration with other health providers (e.g., the medics, the osteopaths, the physical therapists, etc.) is "the wave of the future."

Can you see how Mr. Sosnoski and all the experts in chiropractic are still being held hostage? They are hoping that government entities and insurance providers will include them and begin paying the chiropractors the same fees for services rendered as they pay medical doctors. Nonsense. I have talked with chiropractors who have joined medical groups—some have succeeded, but for the vast majority, it was a nightmare. Chiropractors are treated like red-headed stepchildren and forced to stand at the end of the line. The profession has been doing this for the last eighty years. Where has it gotten us?

Norm Ross's Idea for the Future

I have been involved in chiropractic for fifty-six of my eighty years, and I can attest that nothing has been altered in these fifty-six years. It is mandatory to get the curriculum changed and brought up to modern times by implementing the following:

A) Initiate the 4-3-2 curriculum previously discussed.
B) Encourage chiropractors to get together and create chiropractic malls.

These malls will contain an anchor office (e.g., using a straight adjusting only three-year educated chiropractor that charges affordable fees). This will be the chiropractic volume office. It will see approximately sixty patients per day, five days a week, seeing between twenty-five to fifty new patients per week. This chiropractor will be adjusting the eighteen- to sixty-five-year-old working people who want to get in, get out, and get back to work.

The second office in the mall houses the second tier, chiropractic physician. It is here that women in the profession can excel. We know that the young, the elderly, the chronic, and special needs patients respond favorably to chiropractic care. They do not always need the same type of adjustment that the majority of working people want and need. They need a lighter touch, and this is where specialty adjustments and gentle therapies can be appreciated. I can visualize this being the women's domain where they can become authorities in the care of specialty patients.

The third office can be an oriental medicine/acupuncture office, as many chiropractors utilize this therapy for their patients. Another office could contain a chiropractic physician that specializes in physical therapy, sports injuries, and rehabilitation.

Other offices could include massage therapy, nutritional, and mental health counseling, for example. The idea being that patients primarily begin with straight chiropractic adjustments and move on to other offices as needed.

Today, chiropractors have no apparent place to send 20–30 percent of their patients that are out of their acute treatment parameters. The mall idea is noteworthy because we would no longer have to send these patients back to the medics unless it was an emergency. All these mall offices could feed off of one another. The straight chiropractor in the first office, seeing twenty-five to fifty new patients per week, could keep all the other offices busy. I have used this procedure for the last fifty years. We have seen over 150,000 new patients come through our office. Unfortunately, I've had to send many patients back to the medics because we had no holistic chiropractors who specialized in the chronic, older, and special needs patients, so there was no alternative.

Women of the chiropractic world, can you see this vision of utilizing all the therapies under our current umbrella and branding you as the world's specialist in caring for the young, old, chronic, and special needs patients? In this scenario, the straight chiropractors manually adjust the masses of working folks at affordable cash fees and refer you, the chiropractic physician, the more difficult specialty patients. Naturally, as a specialist, more time will be spent, multiple therapies required, so utilization of insurance for reimbursement and a corresponding fee would be necessary.

This is how insurance should be utilized. As you know, car insurance, house insurance, and most other insurance coverage have a deductible, and insurance is used when you have something costly to recover. Yet in health care, encouraged by the medics (though they will never admit it), insurance coverage for health care became insurance for the sniffles. In fifty years of adjusting, I've found that most low back problems are quickly resolved, similar to a sniffle or the flu, through adjusting. Ninety-five percent of all sniffles or flu will run its course with or without treatment. Most visits to the medic for flu or sniffles are only good for the medics' pocketbook. A lot of insurance money is wasted on those trips.

Perhaps 20 percent of backaches are self-limiting. However, if the other 80 percent can readily get to a straight chiropractor that levels the hips and adjusts the lower lumbar vertebrae thoroughly, they will respond in one to six visits. Many straight chiropractors who specialize in working people do not accept insurance because patients respond rapidly with very little out-of-pocket expense.

In chiropractic's future, we need a two-tiered school, a two-tiered payment structure, and a five- or six-tiered chiropractic mall.

CHAPTER 59

A Little More House Cleaning

We have changed the schools, we have chiropractors adjusting patients when they want and need to be adjusted, you will now be able to distinguish a chiropractor from a chiropractic physician, but there is one item left. Can you afford to go to a chiropractor? Chiropractors will have to change another practice to benefit the public.

Do my fellow chiropractors harbor any guilt from the enormous case fees they collect? Apparently they do not. The profession, as a whole, continues to prey on other's misfortunes. Chiropractors love it when a patient comes in with a problem that has not responded to conventional medical care and therapy. These patients are usually upfront and tell the chiropractor, "Doc, please help me. I will pay you anything if you can get me some help." That opens the lid on Pandora's box because these last hope patients are the ones that will pay upfront for services. Chiropractors are thrilled to have this type of patient walk in the door. It may not be as bad as I paint it because the patient does have an 80 percent chance of getting better. Chiropractors are well known for pulling patients out of some challenging situations and getting their life back on track.

Chiropractic works, and sometimes it takes an extended period to get the body to respond to mechanical alignment. I am not upset with the chiropractor who can take the time, have the patience and perseverance to pull the forgotten medical patient out of the fire. Today the "given up on" patient makes up 20 percent of the chiropractic practice.

Too many chiropractors put every patient that walks through their door into this "forgotten patient" category.

Jason, a thirty-eight-year-old steelworker, got into an awkward heavy lifting situation at work, and the following week went tubing on the lake. These two situations caused his right hip to shift high and inward, giving him considerable grief for two weeks. He went to a nearby chiropractor who informed him after the examination that he could help him. It would require thirty-four visits. If he paid upfront, it would be discounted to $1,500. He walked out without getting any treatment or pain relief. A friend referred him to our office, where we checked and aligned his hips, dropping the right one down and back into place while raising the left to align the hips and level the sacrum. Jason rested twenty minutes, and when he left, his hips were aligned, the sharp pain was gone, and he was ecstatic. It cost him twenty-five dollars for a visit.

When he left, he took a hand full of our cards and said, "You know where I am sending my buddies." We call our new patients after a few days to check on how they responded to the corrections. Jason said he was a little sore the first day at work, but the second day he was great. On the same day that Jason was in our office, we had seen seventeen other new patients. Our chiropractic friend near Jason's house lost a new patient that day. Statistics show that chiropractors average five to six new patients per week. For Jason to fork over $1,500, he would have to have a decidedly compelling reason, and the chiropractor would have to be an exceptional salesperson to pull it off. This, however, is the modus operandi of the chiropractic profession today and may be one of the reasons the profession as a whole is not as successful as it could be.

Chiropractors receive positive feedback from the adjustments they give and the help that patients obtain. This feedback is why the profession can hang on seeing such a small percentage of the population. If we did not get results for the patient, there is no other way chiropractic could stay alive.

Jason's neighborhood chiropractor only needs a few new patients each week to agree to loan him $1,500, and he can make a decent income. Notice he has done nothing yet to earn that money. If the patient quits before the therapy is completed (a lot do because they got better and do not want to spend time going to the chiropractor when they feel well) or they get discouraged because the therapy is not working, that will make room for another chronic patient. Chiropractors will help these chronic, given up on or forgotten patients, and that is terrific. But there is another problem. Chiropractic schools and practice building programs teach students to place every patient in the chronic, given up, on or forgotten patient category. This then leaves out all who should have the right and opportunity to experience periodic structural care and what it can do. Many of you could be responding like Jason but are sitting on the sideline allowed to suffer and degenerate years before your time.

CHAPTER 60

How Can We Get Chiropractic to Succeed?

To begin with, chiropractors could drop the upfront X-ray fee and open their doors to allow people to come and have their spines checked. Chiropractors can buy X-ray machines for less than the cost of a new midsize car, and the supplies are relatively inexpensive. I have not charged for X-rays for the past forty-five years. At a doctor's office, medical clinic, or hospital, you will pay $400, $800, $2,000 or more for -rays. Why are they so expensive? If the X-ray unit and the physical X-rays are manageable, where does the high cost arise? It is from the doctor's expertise. You pay a high fee for medical radiologists to read and interpret X-rays.

After my first couple of years in practice trying to practice as I was taught, selling X-rays, and borrowing money from the patients, I found that I was not a salesman and practice was not enjoyable. I began thinking of the good old days on the farm. On the farm, we had to "give before we got." Living on the farm relied on plowing the ground in the spring, tilling in preparation for planting, planting the seed, cultivating the growing seedlings, watching them mature, and harvesting in the fall. If we had done an excellent job of caring for the plants, we would usually have our reward at harvest time. We did not sell anything in the spring and summer. We spent that time preparing and nurturing the land, which would eventually reward us if we did a good job. My thoughts began leaning toward applying this to my chiropractic practice. I am not a salesman. I am not here to sell people on the idea they need to loan me money. I am here to help people to make them feel better by keeping them in alignment. I have been taught an art form and given a talent that I can share to help others.

I decided to scrap the idea of selling X-rays and begin giving them away. What a difference that made in my practice. It was unbelievable. The pressure was gone. It made practicing fun, and the patients knew they were receiving the care they needed. When you take care of the needs of others, you will never be short of what you need.

Another thing chiropractors could do is to lower their office-visit fee. It has been our practice to follow the local hourly wage that production workers receive in our area. We have a robust, nonunion, industrial base, and wages are presently running twenty to twenty-five dollars per hour. There appears to be a ceiling as to what patients will pay. Once that point is reached, you have to begin selling again. The hourly production wage rate has worked well for us. Even in challenging economic times, we have never had a slow down because we did not overcharge in good times.

Many chiropractors reading this will say, "I will not give my services away!" They must remember they are dealing with an intangible. No chiropractor can guarantee their work nor assure that their adjustment will provide relief. I'm sure they will be pleasantly surprised. They will see a growth in their practice and will find that their income will equal or increase from where they were before lowering their fees. They will be serving more of our fellowmen.

Having a cash practice is much easier when charging an affordable fee. Therefore, many chiropractors may want to get away from accepting insurance and having the hassle of billing insurance carriers. There will be no account receivables and no disputes with patients over money.

Structural analysis exams should start with a history. This history will tell the chiropractor most of what they need to know. For example, a thirty-year-old comes in with a very stiff neck. History reveals that two days ago, he dove into a pool and hit his head on the bottom. X-rays are needed to verify if there is a structural problem that is not an adjustable situation. If a fracture is suspected or found, the patient is sent to the hospital.

On the other hand, a similar thirty-year-old male comes in with stiffness of the neck, and his history shows that he started a new job three weeks ago, which requires him to turn to the right more frequently than his previous position. If there are no other red flags, this patient will be able to accept adjustments and be back in business in no time.

Chiropractors should take any X-rays needed to give them confidence in accepting your case but not merely to charge for that service. Most of the time, for structural alignment of the hips and pelvis, there is no need for a series of expensive X-rays.

The profession is guilty of making all patients take a series of X-rays. With our patient workup, history taking, and palpatory diagnostic skills, there is very little need for everyone to be x-rayed. We have learned a patient management procedure of overcharging once we get a patient in the door by trying to try to extract an X-ray fee from them because they may not come back. We justify any guilt of forcing the patient to buy the X-rays with a fear tactic by saying we do not want to overlook anything. In reality—and I will emphasize this—most of the time, the chiropractor will rapidly peruse the X-ray to see if there are any red flags. They may or may not show them to the patient; they are filed and never looked at again. Sadly, many X-rays taken by chiropractors are primarily used as levers to extract money for a series of visits from the patient when they should be used as a tool to serve the patient better.

Patients often sense that the X-rays are used more like a pawn than a tool. Chiropractors who do not charge for necessary spinal X-rays are appreciated for this token of goodwill that they extend.

When I graduated from chiropractic school fifty-two years ago, we were taught that we should take a full set of X-rays on every patient. It bothered me then and still does as to why we need to take X-rays on each patient when we were taught diagnostic skills that the medic uses. It does not make sense to duplicate the history and palpatory findings with a set of X-rays when we have used standard medical procedures for diagnosis. Fifty years later, we are still trying to prove ourselves, and X-rays are the way chiropractors are saying we know what we are doing.

I'm sure most chiropractors dislike selling X-rays to patients, and I'm sure patients hate having a chiropractor attempt to sell them X-rays.

It becomes a win-win situation for both when X-rays are taken at no charge. All of a sudden, the front door of the chiropractor's office will start swinging off of its hinges. Chiropractors, take whatever view you need and chalk up the cost to overhead. The feeling of freedom is one of the greatest thrills in the world! I will guarantee that if you start giving, and give patients a proper adjustment, the world will beat a path to your door. Giving and getting, it doesn't get any better than that.

To all the chiropractors who are reading this and cannot fathom giving services away. Remember that all patients come to us and walk out of our doors with only a hope and a prayer that the adjustment will give them any relief. There is not a chiropractor in the country that can guarantee their work; they cannot assure that their adjustment will provide relief. Also, there is not a chiropractor in the country who would go to themselves and jump through all the hoops they make you jump through. Most every chiropractor that programs their patients into thirty-four visits/$1,500 cost program are hypocrites, and I will tell you why. When a chiropractor has a problem and they come to me for help (I have had a number do this), if they do not clear up by the third adjustment, they are off to see another chiropractor. Yet they put their patients through a program that they would never agree to themselves. Why do we chiropractors want to be two-faced hypocrites and practice something we would not do or force on our own families? Chiropractors, I implore you to drop your fees and treat people like you would want to be treated. It would create honesty and trust; it would allow us to see a more significant percentage of the population. As for you patients, pray that chiropractors see the light because it is for you that we exist.

Another roadblock for straight chiropractors is the patient's insurance. Get away from billing insurance; all it does is make you dishonest. Lower your fees and let patients pay cash at an affordable price. If you open your door, they will find you and continue to come. At the end of the day everyone has paid and no one owes you anything. We have never sent a bill to any patient in fifty years. There are no account receivables, and we never have to worry about getting into a dispute with a patient over money. Dealing directly with the patient, not promising something we cannot deliver, making it financially feasible for them to pay cash on every visit allows us not to have to deal with insurance.

Essentially every chiropractor in the country using traditional adjusting skills can see sixty patients per day. Usually, it can be done without additional staff. All transactions will be cash or credit cards. No insurance will be accepted; therefore, there are no insurance forms to fill out to take up your time. The chiropractor's adjusting skills will improve when they are concentrating on adjusting patients, and patients sense the improvement in the chiropractor's skills. When care is afford-able and the chiropractor is an excellent adjustor, patients get excited and begin sending their friends and relatives to receive the exceptional care they are experiencing.

Returning to an affordable fee, most people can afford to pay twenty dollars a visit when they need to come. Sixty visits per day times twenty dollars equals $1,200. Working five days a week at $1,200 per day equals $6,000 per week. Making $6,000 per week for fifty weeks equals $300,000 per year. When only one person in a thousand makes $100,000 per year, how special is the chiropractor who can make $300,000 per year by accepting fees the patient can afford? When you do a good job using your talent and skill, it returns dividends. With this in mind, why would the chiropractic profession continue to encourage chiropractors to charge exorbitant fees? Most people could live well on $300,000 per year while improving the health of the world.

CHAPTER 61

Opportunities for All

Today, there are many ways that you can make your money work for you. We have all heard of two ways to make money: (a) you work for your money and (b) you make your money work for you. When I started practice, you could really only invest in real estate or CDs, that was about the extent of it. Today there are countless ways to make your money work for you and your patients as well as the public at large. Just $5,000 will get you into the stock market, and it can occur in your kitchen on your computer. There are many courses available to teach you how to buy and sell in the market.

Chiropractors should learn ways to invest their money and make it work for them. Presently the profession is trying to get rich off the back of their patients. If a chiropractor would open the door to all, make $300,000 a year, and take just $5,000 to put in the market, spending twenty minutes each day on their laptop computer they could become an expert at buying and selling and soon $100,000 could turn into a million dollars.

Another concept is becoming your own banker by using Whole Life Dividend paying insurance. Buying a new car every four years using your own money from your personal bank for forty years could reap additional rewards. Not only would you be driving a new automobile but you could amass $1,500,000 along with a considerable death benefit from the insurance policy.

Why should a chiropractor want to spend time selling patients on care? Even worse, when they have not paid, having to badger a patient to pay what they owe. In my practice, we never have to sell or advertise. We just open our doors, and patients flood into the office. This procedure would allow you to have fun adjusting. It will give you all the time you need to go to your kitchen and make more money than you ever dreamed possible in the stock market or by becoming your own banker through the insurance program. Just think how much you could help worthy causes with your earnings. We need to get into the mainstream and become a class act by being contributors instead of takers in our communities.

CHAPTER 62

Finally

The chiropractic profession has not had any significant changes since its inception, and the adjustment certainly does not need any modification. Recall what Rabbi Lapin stated, "God, nature, and man do not change." Chiropractic is part of the God-nature-and-man paradigm, and it should not change. For example, vertebrae and hips will deviate and compress, vertebrae and hips need to be restored to relieve deviation and compression. This is chiropractic—it is simple, it is vital, everyone in the world should have access to it, and its premise needs no change. However, the current curriculum that educates, trains, and produces the doctor of chiropractic has never been appropriate, and it is an aberration to the universal doctoral format. Below you will find two graphs. The first is the chiropractic doctoral plan, which you will see leads to everything other than specialization. The second is the universal doctoral plan used by all other postgraduate programs. You will observe that it is just the opposite of the chiropractic format. Chiropractic widens the scope and diversifies the courses for their candidates, whereas the mainstream doctoral programs result in specialization when accomplished.

Normal Accepted Doctoral Degree Process

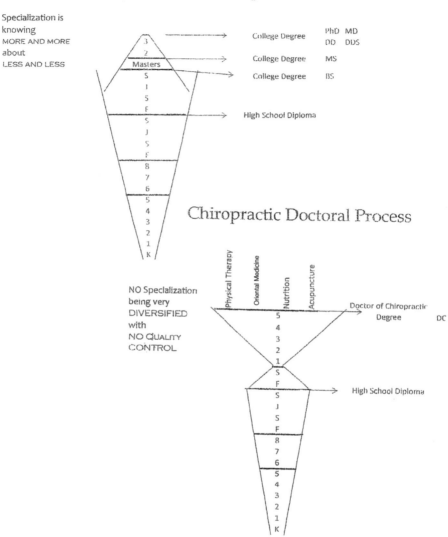

Specialization is
knowing
MORE AND MORE
about
LESS AND LESS

College Degree — PhD MD / DD DDS

College Degree — MS

College Degree — BS

High School Diploma

3
2
Masters
S
1
S
F
S
J
S
F
8
7
6
5
4
3
2
1
K

Chiropractic Doctoral Process

NO Specialization
being very
DIVERSIFIED
with
NO QUALITY
CONTROL

Physical Therapy · Oriental Medicine · Nutrition · Acupuncture

Doctor of Chiropractic
Degree — DC

High School Diploma

5
4
3
2
1
S
F
S
J
S
F
8
7
6
5
4
3
2
1
K

The restructuring of our chiropractic curriculum is an absolute must for chiropractic to function in the mainstream of society. Seeing 5 percent of the population is unacceptable when everyone in the world needs structural attention from time to time.

Restructuring and correcting the curriculum would be very easy and straightforward to accomplish. Several years ago, I showed our chiropractic curriculum to Dr. Jay Thompson, a nationally known curriculum specialist who was reforming the K-12 general education programs for native students in the Aleutian Islands in Alaska. Dr. Thompson was shocked at the formation of our syllabus. It did not take him long to see a myriad of problems too numerous to list that needed to be corrected. He assured me that there are countless curriculum advisors and specialists in mainline education that would be overjoyed to help us set up a proper doctoral program. It would be a feather in any specialist's cap to turn around a great profession and guide it along the appropriate path.

CHAPTER 63

With the Pressure Off

Chiropractic can help change the status of health care of the US and the world if chiropractors will devote their time to adjusting patients. Chiropractors have the philosophy, science, art, and talent in their two hands. All they need is the desire in their hearts to use that knowledge and expertise to help people, and they can become saints.

Danny Thomas, an actor and founder of St. Jude's Hospital, stated, "All of us are born for a reason, but all of us do not discover why. Success in life has nothing to do with what you gain in life or accomplish for yourself. It is what you do for others."

CHAPTER 64

Reformations and Desire

In this treatise, I have given you the history of Chiropractic, along with my experiences in chiropractic. I have given you my thoughts on how to advance chiropractic to reach more suffering patients. To summarize:

1. Changing the curriculum will solve most of the many needed reformations that we have discussed earlier.

   A. Identifying the doctor of chiropractic as the straight chiropractor who will adjust only. They will be known as an adjustment only chiropractor with the designation of chiropractor. Working people will be able to come in and quickly get their hips aligned, sacrum leveled, and spinal vertebra adjusted and not be classified as a chronic condition that requires more care needing an extended range therapy plan. Working people need chiropractors to keep them on the job. They want to come when they need it and get in and get out and get back to work.

   B. Identifying the chiropractic physicians, those who graduated from chiropractic school as a doctor of chiropractic (which allows one to adjust), then continued for two additional academic years to learn ancillary techniques and therapies. Upon graduating with a chiropractic physician degree, they will be better able to concentrate their work on helping medical failures, dismissals and those with chronic conditions

2.   Desire. Do we, as a profession, have the willingness to change?

Do we want to continue on the same track to nowhere? Do we want to continue to kick the can down the road and do nothing? Do we still want to be called quacks and, in some instances, super quacks? Do we sincerely want to help 95 percent of the population? There are masses of people out there that have more faith in us than we have in ourselves. There is a vast population that would love to receive our adjustments and services. Most can neither find a chiropractor, and if they do, they cannot afford them. There are millions of people who do not know we exist and are searching for an alternative. Chiropractic is that alternative. The world needs our services, and they need our adjustments. Join me and help lobby the hierarchy for change. People want our services. They want what we have to offer, and if we can stimulate enough desire to turn this profession around, the term *quack* will readily be transformed into that of *saint*!

Will you please join me in effecting this change?

In humbleness and gratitude,
Norm Ross
Chiropractor

About the Author

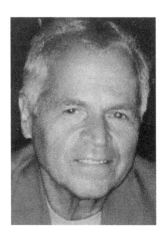

Dr. Norm Ross has a BS in education from Ball State University and taught school for two years prior to entering National College of Chiropractic in 1964. After receiving his doctorate in 1968, he has been in active practice in Northern Indiana for the past fifty-two years, which is nearly 50 percent of the existence of the chiropractic profession.

Dr. Ross has practiced alongside his wife and his brother-in-law, allowing them to have the office open seven days a week. Their mission has been to keep their fees low and affordable. In addition, they accept all patients regardless of condition or ability to pay, creating a haven for many suffering people.

The knowledge amassed from years of adjusting vast numbers of patients has given Dr. Ross exceptional expertise and credence to publish this work.